Relationship Between Health Literacy Scores and Patient Use of the iPET for Patient Education

by

Dr. Melissa A. Sorgeloos

DORRANCE
PUBLISHING CO
EST. 1920
PITTSBURGH, PENNSYLVANIA 15238

Dorrance Publishing Co
585 Alpha Drive
Suite 103
Pittsburgh, PA 15238
Visit our website at *www.dorrancebookstore.com*

ISBN: 979-8-8852-7419-7
eISBN: 979-8-8860-4901-5

Relationship Between Health Literacy Scores and Patient Use of the iPET for Patient Education

Submitted by

Melissa Ann Sorgeloos

A Direct Practice Improvement Project
Presented in Partial Fulfillment of the Requirements for the Degree
Doctor of Nursing Practice

Grand Canyon University
Phoenix, Arizona

May 29, 2019

GRAND CANYON UNIVERSITY

Relationship Between Health Literacy Scores
and Patient Use of the iPET for Patient Education
by
Melissa Ann Sorgeloos

has been approved

May 29, 2019

APPROVED:
Rhonda Johnston, PhD, DPI Project Chairperson
Frances Lorelie Patmon, PhD, Committee Member

ACCEPTED AND SIGNED:

____
Lisa G. Smith, PhD, RN, CNE
Dean and Professor, College of Nursing and Health Care Professions

8/13/2019______________________________
Date

ABSTRACT

Health literacy (HL) can be used as a predictor of health outcomes. Negative health outcomes associated with lower HL levels include barriers to understanding of education materials presented to patients and diminished participation in self-care healthcare behaviors. Nurses, guided by Orem's self-care deficit in nursing theory, can work in conjunction with patients to improve communication through HL assessment. The purpose of this quantitative correlational project was to determine to what degree a relationship existed between health literacy scores, measured with the REALM-SF tool, and patient use of the iPET system to view health education modules for telemetry patients at a 225-bed community hospital in the Southwestern United States. The population was comprised of adult patients ranging from ages 18–89 years old. The sample for this project included 21 adults (N=21) within the age range of 18–89 years old who had been admitted or placed on the telemetry unit as either an observation or inpatient status. Results supported the clinical question as patients that used the iPET for education did score higher on HL assessments by 1.03 points. The correlation between HL and use of the iPET was positive and moderate, $r(19) = .417$, $p = .060$, which sustained the project purpose. Routine HL assessments at the project site are not part of the nursing workflow. Based on HL levels, findings revealed that patients most apt to benefit from use of the iPET did not actually utilize it. Recommendations stemming from this project promote routine nurse assessment of patient HL scores to assure that education materials are presented to patients based upon patient HL levels.

Keywords: Health literacy, patient engagement, healthcare technology, patient education

DEDICATION

I dedicate this project to my mother and father, Karen and Kevin Sorgeloos, both of whom have strongly supported all of my educational endeavors throughout my lifetime. From preschool onwards, my parents have instilled the importance of obtaining an education, while challenging and supporting me to reach for the stars academically. It is not without my parents' love and support that I am in the places I am at today, continually and constantly striving to be the best I can be. As I seek to fulfill my academic dreams, I can only hope my parents realize the impact that their love and support have had on my life. Thank you, Mom and Dad, for planting the seeds and allowing me to flourish.

I also dedicate this project to my wife, Amanda. I would not be at this point of my academic career without her constant love and support. Thank you for believing in me and being there for me—always, every day, and forever.

ACKNOWLEDGMENTS

I wish to express my recognition and gratitude to those who have mentored and supported me throughout this journey to obtain my Doctor of Nursing Practice (DNP) Degree. I cannot express fully, in words, my appreciation and thanks to Dr. Frances Patmon, my content expert/committee member for my Direct Practice Improvement project, whose expertise and knowledge has helped me considerably along my journey. I have learned so much from Dr. Patmon and I greatly appreciate her time and supportive energy. A special thank you to Dr. Katherine Kenny for her support, guidance, and collaboration throughout the various stages of my project. Her time and assistance have had a tremendous impact on me during this wonderful learning experience. I would like to thank Dr. Rhonda Johnston, my committee chair, for all of her feedback and positive support throughout my academic journey. A special thanks to Dr. Herschel Knapp, my mentor from the beginning. I would like to thank Dr. Knapp for all of his time, energy, guidance, recommendations, and helpful advice.

I would like to send wishes of gratitude, thanks, and appreciation to my wife, Amanda, for all of her endless love and support. I could not have gotten through this program without her encouragement. Thank you.

TABLE OF CONTENTS

LIST OF TABLES

LIST OF FIGURES

CHAPTER 1:
Introduction to the Project

Health literacy (HL), within the individual, is defined as the maximum ability that a person has to acquire, comprehend, understand, and utilize necessary health information and services to make healthcare decisions that determine the best individual health outcomes (Centers for Disease Control and Prevention [CDC], 2016). Reaching the attainment of adequate HL and health equity are often impeded by a variety of barriers, which can lead to low HL rates and poor patient health outcomes. Wickham and Carbone (2013) identify low HL as a strong predictor for poor health and negative health outcomes when compared to other demographics such as age, income level, education level, employment status, or race. Negative patient outcomes stemming from lower health literacy levels include improper health maintenance, lack of health prevention interventions, decreased success rates in patient self-management care related to chronic illnesses, and lack of an adequate understanding when following medication prescriptions through adherence or proper use (Wickham & Carbone, 2013). HL levels are noted to be an identifiable risk factor for all-cause mortality rates after making adjustments for age, race, gender, income, education, and health status, causing national concern for the health of the nation (Sudore et al., 2006). HL influences patient understanding of health information, therefore emphasizing the importance placed on the methods for disseminating health education and health information.

Health information is currently presented to patients in a manner that is not easily understood or comprehended by the average person (US Department of Health and Human Services, Office of Disease Prevention and Health Promotion [USODPHP], (2010). Approximately 90% of adults have difficulties utilizing health information that is available via many outlets on an everyday basis (USODPHP, 2010). Additionally, 88% of American adults have some limitation surrounding health literacy, and approximately one-third of Americans have difficulty understanding and comprehending routine health-care-management directions such as following prescription or medication instructions for either themselves or for their family members (Loan et al., 2018). Nursing interventions and nurse participation play an integral role in helping to identify the methods to increase patient participation in their care, through patient engagement, especially when seeking to extract the benefits associated with Health Information Technology (HIT) systems (Patmon et al., 2016). Nurses must account for healthcare technologies when developing patient healthcare plans and health interventions.

It is imperative that nurses adapt to emerging healthcare HIT and integrate workflows to include patient involvement in healthcare technologies, in particular, focusing on the areas involving patient education and patient engagement (Huston, 2013). Low literacy can prohibit proper patient understanding and follow through of behaviors when it comes to nursing educational interventions or uses of technology within an acute setting (Wickham & Carbone, 2013). This DPI project examined the correlation between patient health literacy scores and patient use of healthcare technologies such as the Interactive Patient Engagement Technology (iPET) system. It is important, as nurses, to understand the dynamics between patient health literacy scores and forms of education delivery, so as to better understand and select the best methods available to provide health education to patients, based on varying patient health literacy levels. Delivering healthcare education to patients based on their comprehension capability provides patients with the best opportunity to understand the education material being presented. This aligns with patient engagement and patient inclusion in healthcare decisions, which provides patients the chance to achieve and attain the highest level of understanding and comprehension, while nurses promote positive outcomes and affirmative self-care behaviors for all patients.

This chapter reviews the background behind why this project was selected and presents rationale to back the importance in conducting HL level assessment on all patients. The implications surrounding HL, as it relates to patient use of technology to view health education modules, is presented within the clinical question that guided this project. Supporting information, which emphasizes the significance of the project as it relates to the purpose and pertinence to the advancement of the nursing profession, is presented. Emphases on the importance of nursing interventions as they relate to health education are discussed. The methodology and design used in this project are presented, as well as a definition for the common terms used. Any imperative assumptions, limitations, and delimitations of the project are explained.

BACKGROUND OF THE PROJECT

In the 1990s, there was an increased and heightened global awareness surrounding HL levels in patients, in particular as to how HL related to health education and patient health outcomes (Kutner et al., 2006). Investigators within the United States began to identify the links between patient reading comprehension levels and how it impacted health-related outcomes such as medication adherence, readmission rates, health education, and hospitalization rates (Kutner et al., 2006). In 1995, the United States created the National Health Education Standards to define important guidelines and considerations relative to HL goals on the patient level (IOM, 2004). Once standards were identified, studies surrounding HL sought answers to identify obstacles or issues pertaining to HL, which prevented patients from achieving an optimal understanding of the health information presented. Assessments and surveys were conducted on the national level, to determine the HL statuses of adults within the United States, since barriers and objectives could not be addressed if HL were not known (Kutner et al., 2006).

In 2003, the United States conducted the National Assessment of Adult Literacy. For the first time, the assessment included statistics regarding literacy rates among American adults as they pertained to health literacy (Kutner et al., 2006). The results of the survey revealed that only 12% of the nation was considered to be proficient in health literacy (Kutner et al., 2006). Concerns surrounding the low HL level findings of the 2003 survey, led to the creation of national measures, goals, and guidelines that focused on the best efforts to improve HL rates among adults (Kutner et al., 2006). There have not been any subsequent national HL surveys conducted since 2003 and those results did not account for all of the updates and advancements in health education as they pertain to healthcare technologies, leaving gaps in the measures and goals originally set forth 16 years prior (Kutner et al., 2006). The United States government addressed concerns involving HL and the lack of accounting for HIT.

The most recent Healthy People initiatives lists one of the goals of Healthy People 2020 as to improve the utilization of health communication strategies with HIT to improve population health outcomes and overall healthcare quality while assuring that health equity is achieved and maintained (Office of Disease Prevention and Health Promotion [ODPHP], 2017a). This is important because HIT has the potential to increase patient participation, improve the quality of delivered healthcare, improve patient outcomes, influence patient safety, stabilize healthcare efficiency, and reduce the costs associated with healthcare (Ahlan & Ahmad, 2015). Healthcare clinicians can become more directly connected to patients through health technologies, especially interactive technology devices (Werder, 2015).

Interactive technology devices, such as the iPET system, provides nurses the opportunity to educate patients in the acute care setting through the delivery of health education modules tailored specifically to patients based on their illnesses or disease processes (Patmon et al., 2016). The iPET system provides patients an opportunity to increase their initiative and partake in their healthcare choices through self-directed behaviors such as viewing health education modules tailored to their health maintenance plan (Patmon et al., 2016). To assess patient understanding as it relates to iPET technology, nurses could greatly benefit from obtaining HL levels on every patient (Loan et al., 2018). This would allow for proper nurse assessment of the patient's potential capacity for understanding as well as help nursing identify areas in which the patient may need additional educational intervention considerations (Loan et al., 2018). This DPI project focused on health literacy scores as they related to patient use of technology as a means to obtain educational information in an acute-care setting. Although the literature supports health literacy as it relates to patient outcomes, HIT, and patient education, there are gaps in the literature relative to iPET technologies as a means to view health education and correlations with HL scores.

PROBLEM STATEMENT

It was not known if health literacy scores, measured with the REALM-SF tool, correlated to adult telemetry inpatient use of the iPET to view health education modules when compared to a similar group that did not use the iPET, after both groups of patients were provided the same instructions on functionality and use of the iPET system. Low or inadequate HL is a topic of great concern, as low health literacy levels affect health outcomes on both the national and individual level (Kutner et al., 2006). Studies demonstrate that HL scores can be used to predict patient health outcomes (Rymer et al., 2018) and that health literacy is recognized as a social determinant of health based on patient health outcomes (Logan et al., 2015). There is a noted link between health inequalities with lower HL levels, which are both identified as issues among all population classes (Loan et al., 2018). Noted links are found in greater prevalence among the elderly, the poor, ethnic minorities, and in populations with chronic health conditions (Loan et al., 2018), yet approximately half of Americans fall within a lower HL level category, leaving a large number of individuals as lacking the capacity to comprehend and utilize basic health information that is presented to them (Rymer et al., 2018). This is especially concerning for nurses, who disseminate health education to patients as part of nursing interventions and workflows, often times with education material options being delivered in differing formats, for example electronically, written, or verbally.

One of the nursing goals of patient education delivery is to help the patient engage and actively participate in their healthcare (Feudtner, 2001). Nursing education goals, tailored to the patient individually, are designed to ultimately improve patient health outcomes while improving patient quality of life (Feudtner, 2001). Technological advancements in healthcare can have a direct impact on nursing interventions, especially those involving patient education techniques for the hospitalized patient (Huston, 2013). Using health literacy scores as a predictive factor can help nurses assess to determine a patient's capacity to understand the educational interventions being presented to them, especially as it relates to delivery of information via healthcare technologies (Rouleau, Gagnon, & Cote, 2015). Nurses play an essential role in helping to integrate patient use of iPET technology in the hospital or acute care setting, especially as it relates to the delivery of patient health education information (Patmon et al., 2016). Patients with lower HL scores may have poorer health outcomes and may be less engaged to use technological educational interventions (Mackert et al., 2016).

It would be beneficial to obtain HL levels on all patients to assess the patient's potential capacity for understanding as well as to help nurses identify any areas in which the patient may need additional or different educational interventions and formats. To best understand the impact that HL scores have on patient understanding, assessment of patient HL is imperative (Loan et al., 2018). Knowledge involving HL scores, as it pertains to patient use of iPET technology, was explored in this project so that nurses can better understand the best methods to provide patient health education in the acute setting for patients with varying levels of HL. Although the literature supports HL influences on health education delivery, absent from the literature are studies that assess the extent in which HL scores correlate to or influence patient self-directed use of the iPET system to view educational content through self-controlled, interactive bedside technology systems.

PURPOSE OF THE PROJECT

The purpose of this quantitative correlational project was to determine to what degree a relationship existed between health literacy scores, measured with the REALM-SF tool, and patient use of the iPET system to view health education modules for telemetry patients at a 225-bed community hospital in the Southwestern United States. The independent variable was represented as patient HL scores and the dependent variable was determined by the dichotomous outcome of whether the patient used the iPET to view health education modules, yes or no. All patients were provided the same information and instruction on the functionality of the iPET. HL scores for patients that did use the iPET to view education modules were compared to HL scores for patients that did not use the iPET to view education modules. Discovering whether a correlation exists between health literacy scores and patient use of interactive patient engagement technology to view health education modules is an important consideration for nurses providing care to patients in an acute setting, particularly cardiac telemetry patients. Demographic factors such as age, health status, and ethnicity are linked to health literacy rates (Kutner et al., 2006). Because patients with lower health literacy rates demonstrate mortality rates more than double to patients with higher health literacy rates, nurses must consider assessment of HL levels on all patients (Smith et al., 2018). The patient population for this project comprised of English-speaking adults aged 18 through 89 years of age admitted to a single telemetry unit in a community hospital. Cardiac patients on a telemetry unit were selected because there was an abundance of literature surrounding nurse education delivery on cardiac patients.

Nurses play a central role in the recognition of methods to transform care and create opportunities for improvement in patient outcomes (Institute of Medicine Committee, 2011). HL plays an important part in patient comprehension of the education materials presented in an acute care setting (Loan et al., 2018). This project contributes knowledge to the field of nursing as it seeks to discover if there is a correlation between HL scores and patient use of the iPET to view education material while hospitalized. It is important for nurses to understand the dynamic between patient health literacy scores and patient education, in order to understand the best methods of disseminating health education to patients with varying levels of health literacy and to properly tailor the recommended education type to each patient based on HL levels, so that patients can attain the highest level of understanding to improve self-care behaviors and promote positive patient outcomes (Wittink & Oosterhaven, 2018). Patients may benefit from diverse types of educational materials and not all patients may benefit from education presented through the iPET system at the project site, stressing the importance for nurses to assess the health literacy levels of each individual patient and subsequently deliver targeted education to patients based upon the health literacy levels and recommended education material format with the goals being to improve patient outcomes.

CLINICAL QUESTION

The independent variable was represented as patient HL scores and the dependent variable was determined by the dichotomous outcome of whether the patient used the iPET to view health education modules, yes or no. The lack of a formalized process for nursing units or specialized care areas to routinely screen patients for health literacy levels is problematic, as nursing attempts to delivery patient health education to patients with different levels of health literacy, risking the fact that patients may not understand what is presented to them in the manner it is delivered (Loan et al., 2018). Berkman et al. (2011) found that patients with low health literacy often consume more healthcare resources, highlighting the important need for healthcare systems and nursing to work in conjunction to provide patients with the resources required for targeting the best methods in which to provide patient education to patients based upon patient health literacy levels (Loan et al., 2018). Adoption of a unified form of screening for health literacy has been considered for some time on the national level, yet it has not been completed (Rymer et al., 2018). Since 2012, the Joint Commission has recommended that hospitals assess and document patient health literacy needs, but this recommendation is not a mandate and few healthcare systems have followed this advice (Rymer et al., 2018).

Findings from studies on sites that have implemented the Joint Commission recommendations have demonstrated improved outcomes in patients targeted with several different chronic disease processes (Rymer et al., 2018). Hospitals that routinely screened patients for health literacy demonstrated both lower readmission risks and higher compliance with patient prescribe medication regimens (Rymer et al., 2018). Using health literacy scores as a predictive factor can help nursing predetermine a patient's capacity to understand the educational interventions being presented to them, especially as it relates to delivery via healthcare technologies (Mackert et al., 2016). Concernedly, patients with lower health literacy scores may be less apt to engage in technological educational interventions (Mackert et al., 2016). Nurses proficient in HIT can help patients connect electronically to education modules that can help promote improved healthcare behaviors and improve outcomes during and post-hospitalization (Huston, 2013). Sufficient literature supports the importance of routinely assessing HL as its influence on patient outcomes, education, and patient use of technology are presented. Prior to the completion of this DPI project, it was not known if health literacy scores correlated to adult telemetry inpatient use of the iPET to view health education modules. The following clinical question guided this quantitative project:

Q1: Did adult inpatients (P) that use technologically assisted interactive patient engagement technology (iPET) for health education, (I) versus a similar group that did not use the iPET for health education, (C) show a higher literacy score on the REALM-SF tool (O) when assessed during their hospital stay (T)? The independent variable in this project was represented as patient HL scores and the dependent variable was determined by the dichotomous outcome of whether the patient used the iPET to view health education modules, yes or no.

ADVANCING SCIENTIFIC KNOWLEDGE

The Healthy People 2020 initiative has identified, as one of its goals, the use of health communication strategies and HIT to improve population health outcomes and healthcare quality (Huston, 2013). Health communication and HIT are essential components in shaping societal views on healthcare, as the methods and processes of healthcare information technology create the manner in which both professionals and the public seek, comprehend, and utilize health information (ODPHP, 2017). The way in which this knowledge is obtained and disseminated significantly impacts patient health decisions and actions (ODPHP, 2017). Health decisions, patient self-behaviors, and patient actions are crucial to placate the ongoing patient self-care needs important to the health and well-being of the patient, as identified in the self-care deficit theory of nursing (SCDTN).

Dorthea Orem's SCDTN was used as the theoretical foundation for this DPI project. The SCDTN focuses on the interactions between nurse and patient, so that together, they can assure a clear understanding of what the expectations, benefits, and values are when achieving adequate communication (Orem & Taylor, 2011). Jarvis (2013) finds that technology helps to enhance communication with healthcare workers and improves patient participation in their healthcare choices. The benefits of including patients in their own health-care choices include an increase in patient participation in their own healthcare decisions as well as an increase in patient participation in interventions (Prey et al., 2013). Patient use of the iPET can be a helpful tool to bring patients and nurses together through communication. The iPET system is a patient-controlled aspect of technology that allows patients the ability to utilize the system in a self-decisive and autonomous manner. The iPET system is capable of delivering self-management health interventions to improve patient health communication and health education (Patmon et al., 2016). One of the goals of the iPET system is to improve patient engagement through technology, in the acute healthcare setting (Patmon et al., 2016). To assure patient engagement in iPET use, nurses must assure patients understand the ways in which benefits can be extracted from iPET usage, which can be assessed by several methods, one of which would be to have a pre-working knowledge of patient HL levels.

It is imperative that nurses assess patient levels of understanding when delivering education about technologies, healthcare behaviors, and disease processes (Loan et al., 2018). Patient use of the iPET provides patients with a degree of autonomy, as patients can view prescribed health education modules on their own accord, to enhance patient participation in healthcare education. Providing information on iPET use allows nurses and patients to foster communication. Nurses reported improved levels of communication between patient and nurse after the patient gained some baseline knowledge regarding their illness and disease process by viewing healthcare education modules through the iPET system (Patmon et al., 2016). Prior to the completion of this project, it was not known if health literacy scores, measured with the REALM-SF tool, correlated to adult telemetry inpatient use of the iPET to view health education modules when compared to a similar group that did not use the iPET, after both groups of patients were provided the same instructions on functionality and use of the iPET system. This project will advance population health outcomes by determining if a relationship exists between HL and patient use of the iPET as a self-care behavior. A lower HL score may prevent patients from properly utilizing self-care interventions, such as the use of the iPET to watch prescribed health module videos. If patients are unable to engage in self-care measures, or if one's ability to engage in self-care processes is less than optimal, a self-care deficit would exist, as defined within Orem's SCDTN (Wilson et al., 2003).

SIGNIFICANCE OF THE PROJECT

Individuals with lower HL are less likely to use HIT tools and often perceive them as difficult to use or less useful than traditional means of receiving health information and education (Rymer et al., 2018). Low HL inhibits the patient's ability to comprehend and utilize basic health information presented to patients within a healthcare setting (Rymer et al., 2018). Disparities in access to health information, services, and technology typically yield decreased patient knowledge of chronic disease management and care (ODPHP, 2017a). Additional risk factors related to disparities in access to HIT include adverse outcomes such as higher hospitalization rates and an overall worsening of health statuses and chronic illness processes (ODPHP, 2017a). Accessing HIT and healthcare services has become more complex as technology improves, which has implications on how HL is affected for patients on the individual and population levels (McCormack, Thomas, Lewis, & Rudd, 2016). When considering patient health outcomes and methods to improve patient care in nursing, there must be considerations pertaining to patient communication, HL, and technology.

A National Action Plan exists to improve patient HL and to advance and promote changes in the manner in which health information is communicated (ODPHP, 2017c). This goal ultimately allows patients to make more informed decisions and provides improved access to and understanding of healthcare services and options available for patients (ODPHP, 2017c). Foundational principles of the action plan surmise that all people have the right to health information which allows them to make better-informed healthcare decisions while assuring that healthcare professionals deliver healthcare services in a manner that is concise and clear to promote improved health, longevity, and overall quality of life for patient populations (ODPHP, 2017c). An integral aspect for consideration when delivering patient education includes the evaluation of prior knowledge, cognition status, patient attitudes, motivators, and patient tolerance for errors in treatment approaches (Lessa et al., 2016). Benefits of including patients in their own health decisions include increased patient understanding of healthcare instructions and patient participation in their own care interventions (Prey et al., 2013). Nursing education interventions aimed to improve the patient self-care confidence of heart failure patients promote self-efficacy and improve patient outcomes, have been studied and revealed that heart failure patients have the highest frequency of hospital readmissions in the United States (Baptiste et al., 2014)–. An estimated 25–50% of patients with heart failure will be readmitted to a hospital within 36 months post-discharge (Baptiste et al., 2014). Assessing cardiac patients, and looking at their ability to partake in self-care interventions and patient education programs, has revealed lessened exacerbation of symptoms, lowered readmission rates, and decreased incidence of visits to the emergency department (Baptiste et al., 2014).

This project is significant to both the field of nursing and to the clinical practice site, as the practice site did not actively collect HL data on any patients. Patient participants were selected from one of the telemetry units, as there was sufficient literature to support the various educational techniques involving cardiac patients.

Additionally, there was ample literature noted pertaining to the implementation of technologies in relation to cardiac patient care, interventions, and outcomes. Gaps are noted in the literature, in particular, as they relate to the relationship between HL scores and cardiac patient use of interactive technologies, such as the iPET. Although HIT is readily available to many Americans, it is not readily utilized, most likely because over 50% of American adults fall into a low HL category (Mackert et al., 2016). Prior to the completion of this DPI project, it was not known if health literacy scores, measured with the REALM-SF tool, correlated to adult telemetry inpatient use of the iPET to view health education modules when compared to a similar group that did not use the iPET, after both groups of patients were provided the same instructions on functionality and use of the iPET system. Rymer et al. (2018) find that further studies are necessary to understand the effects that inpatient HL screening can have on the promotion of improved patient outcomes.

In order to understand the effects HL has on cardiac patients and their use of self-driven technologies for educational means, it is imperative that HL levels are measured. Hospitals which routinely screened patient HL levels saw improvements in patient outcomes through improved rates on patient medication adherence and lower readmission rates, yet it was deemed as uncommon for hospitals throughout the United States to actively screen cardiac myocardial infarction patients for health literacy levels (Rymer et al., 2018). After screening HL levels, heart failure patients with lower health literacy levels were discovered to have significantly higher mortality rates that those with higher HL levels (Peterson et al., 2011). These considerations stress the importance that HL may have in terms of patient understanding of education and adherence to care to pertain to cardiac disease processes. Results from this project address gaps and questions surrounding the correlation between HL scores and patient use of interactive technologies that deliver patient education to cardiac patients. The results and findings equate to practical applications which stress the importance of measuring and assessing HL levels on all cardiac patients, as nurses can utilize and apply this information when seeking to deliver health education to patients. HL scores provide nurses with an opportunity to tailor dissemination methods of education materials, based upon HL levels, allowing application of a best-fit format of education material to individual patient needs.

RATIONALE FOR METHODOLOGY

A quantitative methodology was chosen for this DPI project. A quantitative methodological approach for this project was chosen over a mixed or qualitative methodology. Qualitative methodologies focus on the study of people, such as the subjective meaning of experiences to the person, as an individual (McLeod, 2017). Qualitative approaches are focused on the individual and the objectivity of the person (Nieswiadomy, 2012). Qualitative methods seek to understand the social reality of a situation as individuals or groups experience or live it, such as data collected through subjective participant observations or interviews (McLeod, 2017). This project did not focus on seeking patient perceptions of the iPET or concept of HL in a subjective matter; therefore, a qualitative methodological approach was excluded.

Quantitative methodologic approaches are characteristically objective (McLeod, 2017). Quantitative studies consist of data collected via a measurement tool, such as the REALM-SF tool used in this DPI project versus data collected through participant observations or interviews, as would occur in qualitative methodologies in research or studies (McLeod, 2017). Quantitative approaches typically yield data in numerical formats, as it is primarily concerned with measurements (McLeod, 2017). The clinical question for this DPI project asked, do adult inpatients that use interactive patient engagement technology (iPET) for health education, versus a similar group that does not use the iPET for health education, show a higher health literacy score on the REALM-SF tool when assessed during their hospital stay? A quantitative approach best fit the collected variable data sets. The independent variable was represented as patient HL scores and the dependent variable was determined by the dichotomous outcome of whether the patient used the iPET to view health education modules, yes or no. The yes or no response was coded into numerical data for statistical analysis. The project methodology fit within the confines of the project correlational design, which was used to determine if a relationship existed between the two variables of HL scores and patient use of the iPET for education. The project design addressed the connection or importance of the collected quantitative data.

NATURE OF THE PROJECT DESIGN

The design selected for this DPI project was correlational, to align with the project's quantitative methodological approach. This design was chosen over the other available design options since it best addressed the clinical question asking if adult inpatients that used technologically assisted interactive patient engagement technology (iPET) for health education, versus a similar group that did not use the iPET for health education, showed a higher literacy score on the REALM-SF tool when assessed during their hospital stay? The purpose of the project sought to determine to what degree a relationship existed between patient HL scores and patient use of the iPET for education. Price, Jhangiani, and Chiang (2015) define a correlational design as the type of design in which two variables are being measured and assessed to determine the statistical and correlational relationship between them, with little to zero control of the extraneous variables. Correlational designs can also seek to discover if a statistical relationship is casual or purposeful (Price, Jhangiani, & Chiang, 2015).

All patients were administered the REALM-SF tool, and HL scores were assessed on all patient participants. Patient education on the use and functionality of the iPET was delivered to each patient, and teach-back methods were utilized to assure proper communication, and patient understanding of how to use the iPET was achieved. Education was provided through one-on-one instruction with each patient and visual demonstration with each patient handheld device. After the training, all patients were asked to teach-back functionality and use of the iPET. The primary investigator (PI) then left the patient and returned several hours later to, and patients were asked if they used the iPET to view any educational videos. The dependent dichotomous variable outcome revealed whether the patients did or did not use the iPET to view health education modules after being instructed how to do so by the PI through patient yes or no responses.

The independent variable was represented as patient HL scores and the dependent variable was determined by the dichotomous outcome of whether the patient used the iPET to view health education modules, yes or no. During data examination, variable correlation of iPET use was analyzed against the patient health literacy scores. Two groups emerged, patients that did use the iPET for education and patients that did not use the iPET for education. A total of 21 patients participated in this project. Eleven of the 21 patients did use the iPET for education and 10 patients did not use the iPET for education. The correlational design was the best approach to answer the clinical question through the correlation between HL scores and patient use of the iPET for education.

DEFINITION OF TERMS

This section will define health, medical, and variable terms used throughout this chapter. The terms will be defined as used in the context for which they apply to this project. To assure clarification, lay terminology will be used to define terms.

Health Information Technology (HIT). Technology utilized to maintain, store, educate, and analyze health information through an exchange or capacity within an electronic environment (US Department of Health & Human Services [HHS], 2017). Examples of HIT include electronic health records, personal health records, electronic prescriptions, personal health tools, online communities, and interactive patient engagement tools (USA.gov, 2013).

Patient outcomes. Patient outcomes in nursing relate to patient health results as related to nursing care and intervention and are measurable with many variable options (Liu et al., 2014). Examples of patient outcomes include readmission rates, adherence to medications or treatment regimens, patient satisfaction, improvements in conditions, and participation in preventative and wellness self-care behaviors (Charlton et al., 2008).

Patient engagement. Patients are considered engaged when their actions demonstrate an increased interest to improve positive self-care or attain better outcomes through health-promoting actions (Wasson & Coleman, 2014).

Interactive Patient Engagement Technology (iPET). An electronic system with the capability to delivery health system management, communication, education, and distraction services to patients per their control (Patmon et al., 2016). Distraction capabilities of the iPET include relaxation channels and music channels. Entertainment functions of the iPET include on-demand viewing of Hollywood films. Education opportunities allow patients to view specific modules, tailored to patients based on illness or diagnoses (Patmon et al., 2016).

Health literacy. The maximum ability a person has to acquire, comprehend, understand, and utilize basic health information and services to make healthcare decisions that determine the best individual health outcomes (Centers for Disease Control and Prevention [CDC], 2016).

Rapid Estimate of Adult Literacy in Medicine – Short Form (REALM-SF). A tool developed by Dr. Terry Davis. The REALM-SF instrument is considered a valid and reliable measurement tool to effectively and rapidly measure patient health literacy scores (USDHHS, 2016).

Teach-back. Teach-back is a reliable method for nurses to assess patient understanding of health education and occurs when the patient successfully teaches the information back to the nurse by verbalizing, in their own words, their understanding of the instructions or information provided (Badaczewski et al., 2017).

ASSUMPTIONS, LIMITATIONS, DELIMITATIONS

ASSUMPTIONS. The assumptions, limitations, and delimitations present and integral to this project are discussed. The following assumptions were present in this project:

1. It was assumed that participants in this project agreed to do so upon their own free-will and decision. Verbal consent to participate was required from all participants after detailed expectations and explanations of the project were provided to the patient. An IRB approved script was used to provide patients with the proper preliminary information prior to receiving consent from the patient. It was assumed that patients verbally agreeing to participate actually desired to participate in this project and did not feel they were mandated to participate.
2. It was assumed that all patient participants embody an accurate representation of any other current hospitalized telemetry patient, in terms of health status, found within the Southwestern United States. Patient participants were recruited within the telemetry unit, and all patients admitted to the telemetry unit were assumed to have an increased potential for having chronic health conditions versus those from a patient population admitted to another unit

type, such as any other non-specialized nursing unit. This assumption aligned with the heavy focus on cardiac patients and cardiac education associated with this project.

3. It was assumed that patients participating in this project would be honest in their answers. A potential limitation could exist if a patient did not fully understand what was being asked of them, but proceeded to respond to the questions or partake in the project regardless. Assuming that all patients were honest in responses provided, the PI was given the opportunity to conduct data analysis that yielded error-free results which would help answer the clinical question. If patients were assumed to be dishonest with responses, the data collected could not be utilized, since results would yield inaccurate findings upon analysis.

LIMITATIONS. There were limitations in this project. The following limitations were present in this project:

1. A limitation in this project surrounded the patient willingness to participate. Prior to commencing the project, it was assumed that there would be a sample size of approximately 20–50 patients, based on pre-project power analysis calculations. Reaching the high-end targeted sample size of 50 participants was difficult to obtain due to a lack of patient willingness to participate. Difficulties exist in recruiting patients for healthcare related studies, since patients do not place the same importance on scientific relevancy of studies as healthcare scientists place on the study (Sacristán et al., 2016). Some patients play an active role and willingness to participate in healthcare studies, but patient participation is often the exception rather than the norm, despite the essential and imperative need for patient involvement to achieve a complete translation of study findings (Sacristán et al., 2016).
2. Within the confines of the inclusion and exclusion criteria, only patients that spoke and read English could participate in this project. Because the REALM-SF does not have an approved and translatable version in any other language than English, the sample size was limited to include only patients that could read and speak English. This limited the potential sample size by immediately eliminating many patients. Due to the geographical location of the project site, there were many patients on the unit that spoke Spanish, but

were unable to participate in the project due to the exclusion criteria, which was developed, based off of the tool language limitations.

DELIMITATIONS. This project included some delimitations. The following delimitations were present in this project:

1. Patients with health statuses considered as critical in nature, such as patients that are on a ventilator or active breathing assistive device other than oxygen via nasal cannula, were excluded form participation. Patients on a ventilator would not be able to adequately focus on the interventions and questions, putting the patient at risk for harm due to stress and the results of the study at risk for lacking validity. Patients that were sedated were not considered for participation in this project.
2. The exclusion of any patients that were on any form of active isolation precautions was included to assure patient safety and minimize risks. Identified by the telemetry unit charge nurse, any patients that were on isolation precaution measures were not included to participate, even if they otherwise fit the inclusion criteria. The PI adopted, after inclusion and exclusion criteria were set, to exclude any isolation precaution patients to preserve patient safety and minimize all patient risks.

SUMMARY AND ORGANIZATION OF THE REMAINDER OF THE PROJECT

Health literacy refers to the ability a person has to understand, utilize and consume health information presented to them as delivered through a variety of differing methods (CDC, 2016). Health literacy can be used as a predictor of health outcomes (Rymer et al., 2018). Patients with lower HL levels are expected to demonstrate less favorable patient outcomes than patients with higher HL scores (Wickham & Carbone, 2013). Using health literacy scores as a predictive factor can help nursing predetermine a patient's capacity to understand the educational interventions being presented during educational intervention, especially as it relates to information delivery via healthcare technologies (Rouleau, Gagnon, & Cote, 2015). Patients with lower HL scores may be less engaged to participate in self-driven technological educational interventions (Mackert et al., 2016).

Dentzer (2013) defines patient engagement as the behaviors and actions patients take towards their health. Patient engagement has been identified as an integral aspect of nursing care to help improve patient experiences, patient satisfaction, and patient outcomes (Patmon et al., 2016). Studies have demonstrated that using HIT, to increase patient engagement, could result in positive patient outcomes (Patmon et al., 2016). Although low health literacy is prevalent among all ages, all ethnicities, and all socioeconomic classes, well-established links exist between health inequalities and low HL among particular populations, such as the elderly, the poor, ethnic minorities, and in populations with chronic health conditions (Logan et al., 2015). Healthcare organizations have begun implementing HIT to engage both patients and caregivers in the acute clinical setting (Dalal et al., 2016). Implementing health information technologies in the acute clinical setting will not only engage patients and increase their interest and participation in their own health choices but also hope to improve patient self-care and self-management in a manner that results in favorable patient outcomes (Dalal et al., 2016).

Technology is considered a crucial aspect to bridge gaps as they relate to HL and patient health outcomes. Technology has become interwoven into healthcare delivery and design, in many forms, and is used in many different areas of healthcare and nursing. Although there are many examples of technologies used within nursing and healthcare, those of particular interest provide patients targeted information by standardizing educational messages within a program that can be tailored to meet individual patient needs, based upon specific illness or disease processes (Wickham & Carbone, 2013). The iPET, used as the interventional piece in this project, is a technology system that delivers a multitude of interventional options for patients (Patmon et al., 2016). Nursing interventions as related to the educational aspects of the iPET system were of particular importance in this project.

The identified nursing intervention of this project was the delivery of instruction to the patient on the educational aspects of the iPET. Although the iPET is an intervention in itself, not all patients would use the iPET, even though it was presented to them. Providing instructions on iPET use and functionality was chosen as a means of intervention, as research demonstrates that use of patient engagement technology can help improve patient outcomes and health literacy levels influence patient outcomes (Patmon et al., 2016). Prior to the completion of the project, it was not known was if health literacy scores, measured with the REALM-SF tool, correlated to adult telemetry inpatient use of the iPET to view health education modules when compared to a similar group that did not use the iPET, after both groups of patients were provided the same instructions on functionality and use of the iPET system.

When looking at patient perspectives regarding patient HL and use of interactive engagement technology, it is important to understand the effect that patient HL scores have on the use of the iPET for education, the patient population selected for this project was based on existing research regarding patients living with chronic cardiac health conditions. Literature demonstrated that patients with cardiac conditions had lower readmission rates when patients participated in their own healthcare learning (Riley, 2015). Lessa et al. (2016), Baptiste et al. (2014) and Riley (2015) all stressed the importance of early patient educational nursing interventions during admission in the acute setting for heart failure patients. Health literacy and poor health outcomes are linked and more prevalent in populations with chronic health conditions (Logan et al., 2015). Measuring health literacy levels was a key aspect of this DPI project.

Assessing routine or standardized patient HL rates were not routinely collected at the project site; therefore, there was no existing health literacy data for the population served at project site. A lack of existing HL rate data within this population allowed this project to gain insight regarding HL scores and how they have an effect on patient use of the iPET for health education in patients with chronic health conditions. Patients admitted to a telemetry unit were assumed to have an increased potential for having chronic health conditions versus those from a patient population admitted to a general, non-specialized, nursing unit. Assumptions were based upon literature regarding cardiac readmission rates and the importance of self-care behaviors in the treatment of heart failure (Kollia, Giakoumidakis & Brokalaki, 2016). Consequently, it is imperative that patients with low HL levels are identified during hospitalization, so that the nurses delivering health education and teaching to patients can assure properly tailored interventions are utilized to educate patients.

Nursing plays a crucial role in helping patients understand, foster, and enhance HL (Loan et al., 2018). Patients can use the iPET for education to enhance healthcare promotion and improve self-care behaviors for a range of chronic and acute disease states. Depending upon the patient's illness or disease state, patients could view videos on the iPET that cover surgical wound care, the measurement of daily weights for congestive heart failure patients, monitoring glucose levels, routine self-care concerns, readmission prevention, and the importance of medication adherence (Patmon et al., 2016). Without working knowledge of patient HL levels, nurses cannot properly assess if formats, such as the iPET, are most fitting for the patient. Nursing interventions, enhanced through technologies like the iPET systems, can be used to improve patient and nurse communication and can impact nursing interventions related to the delivery of patient healthcare education. Patient health literacy levels in the form of numerical data were obtained. Patient health literacy scores, obtained from the REALM-SF were collected on every patient; scores for those who used the iPET system were compared to those who did not use the iPET system. Numerical data, such as the patient HL scores, was applicably analyzed through quantitative correlational approaches.

Chapter 2 will present a review of current evidence surrounding patient education, HL levels and patient use of technology. Chapter 3 will describe the methodology, project design, and procedures for this project. Chapter 4 will detail how the data was analyzed and provides both a written and graphic summary of the results. Chapter 5 will grant an interpretation and discussion of the results, as they relate to the existing body of literature related to health literacy scores, patient use of technology, the promotion of patient engagement, and patient self-care behaviors.

CHAPTER 2:
Literature Review

The purpose of this quantitative correlational project was to determine to what degree a relationship existed between health literacy scores, measured with the REALM-SF tool, and patient use of the iPET system to view health education modules for telemetry patients at a 225-bed community hospital in the Southwestern United States. Approximately 77 million American adults are not able to effectively understand healthcare instructions, making it difficult for the average American to make the most optimal and informed healthcare decisions (HHS, 2008). Healthcare systems and clinicians play a vital role in assessing HL, as they work in conjunction with patients to educate and analyze the patient understanding of healthcare education materials (HHS, 2008). It is important that patients with low HL levels are identified while hospitalized and preferably early in the admission process (Lessa et al. (2016), so that the nurses can assure interventional educational materials are presented in the correct format to reach patients levels of comprehension, as determined by HL scores. This review deliberates the importance of nurses screening HL as it pertains to patient use of interactive technologies that promote patient engagement, which subsequently leads to the most optimal patient outcomes.

The theoretical foundation used for this DPI project was Dorthea Orem's self-care deficit theory of nursing (SCDTN). Applicability of the SCDTN as it relates to the DPI project is described within this chapter. SCDTN application precedes the literature review section of this chapter. Seminal research articles, systematic reviews, scholarly journal articles, evidence-based research, randomized control trials, observational studies, and case reports on HL, patient education, health information technology, and iPET systems were acquired from databases including PubMed, Cochrane Library, CINAHL, Up-to-Date, ClinicalKey, Medline, US National

Library of Medicine and AccessMedicine. Medical Subject Headings (MeSH), keywords and search terms used to access literature applicable to this project included HL, patient education, patient outcomes, patient engagement, health information technology, teach-back, nursing education interventions, technological impact on patients, evaluating and measuring HL, nursing health promotion, technological impacts on nursing, nursing technologies, patient health technologies, interactive patient technologies, nurse and patient communication, HL concerns, and Dorthea Orem. The study was appraised and synthesized in this review and study purposes, samples, methodologies, and findings are discussed.

This chapter includes background information as it relates to the problem and an extensive review of the literature regarding the major themes of HL, HIT, patient education, and the iPET system. Heavy emphasis was placed on the major themes and subthemes. Subthemes within this review include HL measurements and evaluations, health literacy outcomes, national considerations for HL, health literacy nursing considerations, the teach-back method, patient engagement, and interventional aspects of the iPET. The theoretical foundation, which supported this project, are covered in detail. HL, as it relates to health education and patient outcomes are discussed as pertinent to large population, such as on a national level, down impacts on the individual patient level.

In the 1990s, health literacy, health education, and patient outcomes became a topic of national discussion (Kutner et al., 2006). During that time, global awareness began to increase, especially pertaining to how education was linked to health and health outcomes (Kutner et al., 2006). Global studies had started demonstrating both meaningful and measurable benefits relating to educational interventions and their correlation on patient outcomes (Kutner et al., 2006). American investigators began to explore the links between reading skill levels with an array of health-related outcomes, which included health knowledge, medication adherence, hospitalization and readmission rates (Kutner et al., 2006).

In 1995, the Joint Committee on National Health Standards published a set of standards on optimal methods to achieve adequate HL within the United States (IOM, 2004). Achieving Health Literacy was one of the subtitled sections to the National Health Education Standards. These standards described the necessary knowledge and skills considered essential to HL, at that time (IOM, 2004). The standards, which provided a framework for health education curriculum, detailed the recommendations of what students should know about health education at the end of fourth, eighth, and eleventh grade (IOM, 2004). Studies in subsequent years determined that these standards were not being met, placing heavy emphasis on deciphering and determining what the barriers and obstacles were which prevented these recommended standards from being achieved.

Findings from studies conducted at that time determined that health professionals had limited education in HL and lack proper training on what health literacy was as well as the importance HL had on patient outcomes (IOM, 2004). Due to the limited foundation of HL knowledge, methods and ideas dealing with how to develop and improve HL skills for patients was lacking (IOM, 2004). Opportunities to measure HL levels required the implementation of interventions within existing adult education programs as well as those within the health community (IOM, 2004). The desires to integrate adult learning programs with health community partnerships were noted in studies conducted at that time (IOM, 2004). Studies conducted began to note known barriers preventing the achievement of successful HL levels within the elementary and upper-level education systems, ranging from kindergarten through twelfth grade (IOM, 2004).

The IOM (2004) sought to build upon the lack of such underdeveloped elementary programs, in an effort to improve HL within the United States. The IOM (2004) developed a vision to create a health-literate America, indicating the importance of improving the health of individuals and populations, as they attempted to improve HL at the elementary and adult levels. In 2004, it was discovered that additional learning was necessary as it pertained to the causal pathways between patient education and health outcomes, including the roles literacy plays, as well as how HL contributes to patient health and health outcomes (IOM, 2004). It was deemed necessary to assess the HL levels on a national level.

In December of 2005, the first reports of the 2003 National Assessment of Adult Literacy (NAAL) were released, providing the United States with the first measurable data about HL rates of adults across the nation (Kutner et al., 2006). The 2003 survey found that only 12% of the nation tested as being proficient in health literacy (Kutner et al., 2006), revealing that approximately 77 million American adults are not able to effectively understand healthcare instructions, making it too difficult for the average American to make the best healthcare decisions (HHS, 2008). Results from the 2003 NAAL were crucial to the development of HL studies and measures that followed in subsequent years. Limitations from the NAAL study continue to exist, as no other extensive HL study has been completed on a national level in the last 16 years (Kutner et al., 2006).

At the time of the NAAL study in 2003, health literacy measurements only focused on health-related written or printed educational materials, not accounting for technology integration or other methods of disseminating education materials to patients (Kutner et al., 2006). This is troublesome when trying to apply the findings nearly two decades later, especially since technologies in healthcare have advanced considerably over the past 16 years. HL levels may have increased or decreased as a result of the integration of technologies, but these results are not known. HL, patient outcomes and patient engagement are measured through smaller-scale studies, with pertinent findings reported. Patients engaged in their healthcare have higher levels of patient satisfaction, increased comprehension of their overall plan of care, better participation in health improving behaviors and improved overall health and outcomes (Prey et al., 2013). Huston (2013) found that nurses need to adapt to the emerging healthcare HIT and must learn to include the patient in healthcare technologies, in particular, focusing on the areas involving patient education and patient engagement.

It is estimated that 71% of American adults have used the internet to search for health information, with approximately 21% having used a form of technology to track health information (Wickham & Carbone, 2013), yet patients are still lacking the necessary HL comprehension to understand presented health materials (Loan et al., 2018). The Office of Disease Prevention and Health Promotion (ODPHP) lists one of the goals of Healthy People 2020 as improving the utilization of health communication strategies with health information technology (HIT) to improve population health outcomes and overall healthcare quality while assuring that health equity is achieved and maintained (2017a).

Healthcare providers and nursing, over time, will become more directly connected to patients through interactive technology devices (Werder, 2015). HIT demonstrates many benefits as it relates to patient outcomes, in particular the potential to increase patient participation, improve quality of healthcare, improve patient outcomes, influence patient safety, stabilize healthcare efficiency, and reduce the costs associated with healthcare (Ahlan & Ahmad, 2015). As technologies continue to emerge, trends involving integration into nursing workflows and patient use of technologies through patient engagement will continue to be explored (Prey et al., 2013). Nurses proficient in HIT can help patients connect electronically to education modules that will help promote improved healthcare related behaviors and improve positive outcomes post hospitalization (Huston, 2013).

Patients engaged in their healthcare have higher levels of patient satisfaction, increased comprehension of their overall plan of care, better participation in health improving behaviors and improved overall health and outcomes (Prey et al., 2013). Nursing participation, through communication and interventions, play an integral role in helping to identify the methods that can increase patient participation in care, through patient engagement, especially while extracting the benefits associated with using Health Information Technology (HIT) systems (Patmon et al., 2016). The iPET system is an interactive patient engagement technology that provides patients an opportunity and initiative to partake in their healthcare choices through self-directed behaviors such as viewing health education modules tailored to their illness and health maintenance plan (Patmon et al., 2016).

Nursing could greatly benefit from obtaining HL levels on every patient, to assess the patient's potential capacity for understanding as well as help nursing identify areas in which the patient may need additional educational intervention considerations (Loan et al., 2018). This DPI project focused on health literacy scores as they related to patient use patient use of technology to obtain educational information. Nursing plays a crucial role to help foster and enhance patient HL (Loan et al., 2018). Nurses play an essential part in helping integrate patient use of iPET technology in the hospital or acute care setting, especially regarding the delivery of patient health education (Patmon et al., 2016). Since there is no literature related to patient use of the iPET as it compares to HL and the project site does not currently assess HL scores on its patients, there are gaps in the literature pertaining to correlation of HL scores as they relate to patient use of the iPET system for educational purposes.

THEORETICAL FOUNDATIONS

Orem's SCDTN provides the theoretical foundation for this DPI project. Orem's SCDTN can be applicable to fit the dominant aspects of any nursing practice situations (Orem & Taylor, 2011). Orem identified the SCDTN as a general theory, applicable to all nursing scenarios (Fawcett, 2003). Since the SCDTN is considered applicable to all nursing situations, it is not just considered applicable to an individual patient scenario, rather can be applied to groups and populations (Fawcett, 2003). The SCDTN focuses on the interactions between nurse and patient, to determine a clear understanding of what the qualitative and quantitative values are between variables of both the patient and the nurse during healthcare nurse and patient interactions, but can be applied to the overall communications between nursing and population groups (Orem & Taylor, 2011).

The SCDTN has progressed over the decades since its formation, with early foundations of the theory first being formulated in the 1950s (Banfield, 1998). Widely used as a theoretical framework in nursing studies, the SCDTN was found to be most applicable for use in correlational, case study, and quasi-experimental methods of investigative projects (Banfield, 1998). This DPI project utilized a correlational design, which is applicable to fit within the SCDTN. Orem explained that early concepts of the theory focused on understanding the complexities of nursing as a profession, yet later attention was given to the recognition of nursing and the complexities of the interactions between nurse and patient (Orem & Taylor, 2011). The foundation of Orem's theory holds that humans own the ability and capacity to complete deliberate and necessary self-care actions, known as the person's self-care agency (Orem, 1995). It is the self-care agency that motivates patients to partake in healthcare-related decisions and engage in communication with healthcare providers and nurses.

Within the self-care agency, the patient holds self-care abilities that influence both internal and external behaviors and it is these behaviors which allow patients to complete self-care tasks (Villarruel et al., 2001). Per the SCDTN, self-care behaviors are necessary to satisfy the continual and ongoing self-care needs that are vital to a person's health and well-being (Villarruel et al., 2001). Orem asserts that external factors, such as age, gender, and sociocultural statuses can impact and influence self-care agencies (Villarruel et al., 2001). External factors, such as patient health literacy levels, can impact and influence self-care agencies (Chen et al., 2012). As HL levels impact comprehension, self-care deficits can occur when there are weaknesses regarding HL statuses.

Orem finds that a lack of information, a lack of comprehension, or any limited judgment with decision-making abilities is considered a barrier and limitation to self-care, as it interferes with any potential deliberate action towards self-care (Orem, 2001). If nursing is aware of potential barriers, prior to delivering education on self-care techniques or healthcare behaviors, barriers could be addressed properly, allowing patients to fully understand and comprehend what is being taught to them or, at minimum, provide them the confidence and desire to want to participate in self-care. The importance of assessing and measuring the patient's ability to understand and comprehend can foster assurance that patients will be able to effectively partake in self-care behaviors, as patients must be able to comprehend what is being taught to them before they can properly apply the information to self-care behaviors or actions (Orem, 2001).

Nursing interventions, such as guiding, directing, educating, teaching, and providing physical or emotional support, are vital components to nursing functions pertinent to addressing patient self-care deficits (Orem, 1995). Orem's theory supports nursing goals as they relate to assisting patients to meet required needs for care (Villarruel et al., 2001). Nurses can utilize several interventional means in order to help guide patients that need assistance when it comes to self-care deficits or needs (Villarruel et al., 2001). Assessment of HL levels and providing the education, guidance, and direction for patient use of the iPET functions were both performed in this project. In an effort to obtain knowledge regarding HL scores and patient self-care behaviors, the purpose of this quantitative correlational project was to determine to what degree a relationship existed between health literacy scores, measured with the REALM-SF tool, and patient use of the iPET system to view health education modules for telemetry patients at a 225-bed community hospital in the Southwestern United States.

Major concepts within Orem's SCDTN include the patient's ability to engage in self-care activities, patient background, patient health status, and the patient's therapeutic self-care demand, which consists of the quantity of activities that are necessary to meet a patient's requirements for self-care (Wilson et al., 2003). This

DPI project assessed the patient's HL status through the REALM-SF tool, as a means to correlate the score with patient use of the iPET, to determine if HL levels influence the patient's ability to engage in self-care activities, such as using the iPET to view prescribed healthcare education modules. Patient background and health statuses were assessed with the assistance of the unit charge nurse when applying project inclusion and exclusion criteria. Patient diagnoses were not known to the PI, but demographic background data such as gender and estimated age was collected during the interview with the patient. The patient's self-care demand was determined when following up with the patient to determine if the patient utilized the iPET, yes or no, to view health modules.

The SCDTN was used as a foundational guide to answer the clinical question. The clinical question asked, did adult inpatients that used technologically assisted interactive patient engagement technology (iPET) for health education, versus a similar group that did not use the iPET for health education, show a higher literacy score on the REALM-SF tool when assessed during their hospital stay? Patient use of the iPET for education, the dependent variable, allowed patients to exercise autonomy, as patients had complete control of whether they were able to view the prescribed health education modules at a self-determined pace. Assessing patient levels of understanding through assessment of the independent variable of HL is imperative, especially when delivering education about healthcare and disease processes. According to the SCDTN, nursing actions, such as guiding, directing, educating, teaching, and providing physical or emotional support, are vital components to nursing functions pertinent to addressing patient self-care deficits, which may be present because of patient low HL levels. Patients may feel inadequate, embarrassed, or incompetent because they do not understand or comprehend the directions or education presented to them (Chen et al., 2012). When patients lack confidence, such as with low HL, patients are less likely to adhere to health promoting behaviors and self-care actions, causing a deficit in self-care (Chen et al., 2012). Patients with a self-care deficit may not be able to fully understand education materials, making it important to ascertain the reasons why a patient may or may not use the iPET to view educational videos. It is necessary to determine if patients may be at risk for deficits in self-care and one method to assess this would be to assess HL scores on all patients and determine which patients used the iPET for education.

It was not known if health literacy scores, measured with the REALM-SF tool, correlated to adult telemetry inpatient use of the iPET to view health education modules when compared to a similar group that did not use the iPET, after both groups of patients were provided the same instructions on functionality and use of the iPET system. If patients are unable to engage in self-care measures, or if one's ability to engage in self-care processes is less than required, a self-care deficit would exist (Wilson et al., 2003). A lower HL score may prevent patients from properly utilizing self-care interventions, such as the use of the iPET to watch prescribed health module videos, yielding to a self-care deficit for the patient.

Under Orem's theory, nursing aims to assist all persons in need of achieving self-care. This would include the recognition and addressing of the internal and external factors that may inhibit a patient from addressing self-care deficits or needs. The ultimate goal of nursing, under the confines of the SCDTN, is to recognize a deficit and assist in the necessary manners to help the patient improve self-care behaviors. It is important for nursing to understand the dynamic between patient HL scores and patient use of the iPET for education, so as to understand the best methods to provide patient health education to patients with varying levels of HL. Noting the patient HL scores helps nursing identify a potential self-care deficit, allowing nurses the opportunity to intervene through education and discussion, which can help influence the factors that could help improve a patient's self-care agency and increase engagement. Nurse assessment and intervention can begin early in the nurse-patient relationship.

Delivering patient education early in the admission process demonstrates positive patient outcome results (Lessa et al., 2016). Kollia, Giakoumidakis and Brokalaki (2016) stress the importance of self-care in the treatment of heart failure. Patient involvement in their care, through self-care behaviors has an impact on patient outcomes. Important education provided to heart failure patients during the admission process, such as the necessity of monitoring daily weights, the importance of fluid restrictions, the significance of physical activity, adhering to medication therapy, and the signs and symptoms of decompensation, demonstrated positive results in terms of readmission levels and mortality rates (Lessa et al., 2016). The literature is plentiful as it relates to HL, cardiac patient education, patient engagement, and HIT.

REVIEW OF THE LITERATURE

An extensive and thorough review of the literature will be presented as it pertains to the major themes of HL, HIT, iPET, and patient education. As outlined in the introduction section of this chapter, the major themes and subthemes. Subthemes within this review include health literacy measurements and evaluations, health literacy outcomes, national considerations for health literacy, health literacy nursing considerations, the teach-back method, patient engagement, and interventional aspects of the iPET are reviewed and discussed.

HL was explored as it is relative to the importance of patient outcomes and national concerns. The National Academies of Sciences, Engineering, and Medicine (NASEM) (2015) define health literacy as the capacity to which an individual is capable of obtaining, processing, and comprehending basic health information or services, to make decisions about their healthcare. Patient health literacy considerations involve adapting a multidimensional approach, as health literacy encompasses consideration for the cognitive, social, and navigational skills of each patient (Lambert & Keogh, 2014). In 2003, the United States conducted the only national study to date on the nation's HL status, which found only 12% of the nation tested as being proficient in health literacy (Kutner et al., 2006). Healthcare systems and clinicians play a vital role in assessing HL levels and identifying barriers in HL, as they work in conjunction with patients to educate and analyze the patient understanding of healthcare education materials (HHS, 2008).

HEALTH LITERACY

If an official HL measurement tool is lacking, the teach-back method can be used to help nursing assess and discover any misunderstandings or miscommunications with the patient (Ingram & Kautz, 2018). The teach-back method is a reliable and promoted technique often used as a means for healthcare providers to assess patient understanding through communication feedback. The teach-back technique occurs when the nurse has the patient verbalize in their own words, their understanding of the instructions or information provided through nurse-to-patient education (Badaczewski et al., 2017). The teach-back method is promoted by the American Academy of

Pediatrics, American Medical Association Foundation, and Joint Commission as a means to communication effectively to improve patient adherence to treatment plans while protecting patient safety (Badaczewski et al., 2017).

Measurement and evaluation. There are a variety of valid and reliable tools available to measure patient health literacy (Alqudah, Johnson, Cowin, and George, 2014). Alqudah et al. (2014) conducted a study to analyze the various available tools to measure HL and find which one would be most suitable for use by emergency room nurses. This study had especially important considerations since time is a valuable consideration in the emergency department. The purpose of the study was to determine which tools were considered valid and reliable while best fitting the fast-paced environment of an emergency room. Features of the available tools were considered, including the advantages and disadvantages of each tool, the reliability, and validity of each tool, and the time it took to administer and score the patient's HL. Because there are so many tools available, three particular criterion were applied to all instruments considered: tools that use word recognition procedures, tools that take no longer than five minutes to administer and score, and tools that have demonstrated correlation with their counterpart tools, such as those that demonstrate concurrent validity with other related tools, for example the Rapid Estimate of Adult Literacy in Medicine-Short Form (REALM-SF) with its parent, the Rapid Estimate of Adult Literacy in Medicine (REALM).

Tools that demonstrated the shortest time to administer included the Newest Vital Sign (NVS), the REALM-SF, and the Wide Range Achievement Test-Revised (WRAT-R) or WRAT version 3 (WRAT-3). The methodology of the study was achieved through database searches of English written articles published between 1990 and 2011. The high patient turnover rate and fast-pace of the emergency room were considered when isolating appropriate tools.

The WRAT-3 tool, used to measure HL, was designed to measure basic reading skills, spelling, and mathematics of general literacy skills (Alqudah et al., 2014). The WRAT-3 tool is the oldest and second most commonly used tool to measure the HL of both patients and caregivers. The tool can be administered to patients aged five to 74 years old. There are two sections to the tool, a letter test, and a word portion. The letter section asks patients to pronounce 15 letters, and the word section asks the patient to pronounce 42 words aloud, with the word arrangement flowing in ascending order according to word difficulty. The WRAT-3 test takes three to five minutes to administer. Concurrent validity of the tool and strong correlations are noted when compared to the California Test of Basic Skills and the Stanford achievement test with 0.72 and 0.87 scores. The WRAT-3 test has shown high test-retest reliability (Alqudah et al., 2014).

The REALM-SF was noted to be the most usable form of tools found within prior medical studies, especially in healthcare settings, as its context pertains to health-related items (Alqudah et al., 2014). The REALM-SF tool shows high concurrent validity with its parent, the REALM tool. The REALM has demonstrated high test-retest reliability at $r = 0.97$ and $p = <.001$. The REALM-SF tool contains a list of seven basic medical terms (Alqudah et al., 2014). Patients are asked to read each word aloud to the interviewer, earning a score of one when pronounced correctly within a five second period. Words that are not correctly pronounced or that take a patient longer than five seconds to verbalize are given a score of zero for that word (Alqudah et al., 2014). Patients may skip or pass on a word, which would equate to a zero score for that word. The level of health literacy is determined based on the total score of the words.

A score total of zero to three equates to inadequate or low health literacy (Alqudah et al., 2014). A score of four to six equals marginal HL, and a score of seven indicates adequate HL. The REALM-SF test has been validated and tested on different age groups. The advantages of using this tool include the short amount of time it takes for patients to complete, but one of the noted limitations is that the results do not account for grading HL levels beyond a ninth grade reading level (Alqudah et al., 2014).

Alqudah et al. (2014) discussed the NVS tool. The NVS tool is available in both English and Spanish (Alqudah et al., 2014). With the NVS tool, patients are asked to answer six questions based off of information provided on a nutrition label. Questions are scored as being either correct or incorrect and tallied to score with results of four or more correct responses as equating to adequate literacy, a score of three equaling marginal literacy, and scoring a two or less as demonstrating inadequate literacy. The NVS demonstrated strong correlation and sensitivity with the Test of Functional Health Literacy in Adults (TOFHLA), with a Cronbach's a = 0.76 (Alqudah et al., 2014).

The results of the study found that the REALM-SF tool was the best approach for nurses working in an emergency department (Alqudah et al., 2014). The REALM-SF was noted to be used successfully within the emergency setting and allowed for a quick and efficient method to identify patient HL levels. It was noted that further studies are recommended to target usage by varied age groups. Conclusions of the study identified the REALM-SF as a simple and swift tool to measure HL in a fast-paced clinical setting, as it can be administered in less than one minute.

Huang et al. (2018) conducted a study which aimed to explore the factor structure of the NVS tool, commonly used to measure HL. The study considered the concepts which explore how identifying the factor structure could help healthcare providers choose appropriate interventional strategies to address patient HL concerns, to improve overall health outcomes. The NVS survey was designed as a quick measure to formulate a numerical HL score based on the response to a series of six questions which relate to information printed on a nutrition label from a container of ice cream (Weiss et al., 2005). The patient reviews the nutrition label while responding to the six questions asked by the interviewer.

Huang et al. (2018) used a cross-sectional design study. The NVS tool was administered to patients at two family medicine clinics within the United States. Patient participants were at least 20 years old and all were diagnosed with type 2 diabetes. Participants were prescribed at least one oral antidiabetic medication, and all spoke English as a primary language. Results indicated that 57% of participants were female. The mean age of participants was 58.7 years old. Of the overall 174 qualified participants, 118 patients were Caucasian, and 43 were African-American. 62% of the participants reported having attended college at some level. Discussion findings recommended strategies to improve patient comprehension of health information, which included revisiting and reiterating key aspects of patient self-care techniques, confirming patient understanding of education via the teach-back method, and using pictorial images and shapes as necessary in pamphlets and education materials. Conclusions of the study found that the numeracy and document literacy both adequately represent the factor structure of the NVS tool and can be utilized to assess health literacy in greater detail on patients that have type 2 diabetes.

Shigaki, Kruse, Mehr, & Ge (2012) conducted a study comparing the REALM tool with the NVS tool to measure HL in patients with diabetes. Both the REALM and NVS are the most commonly used tools to measure HL in healthcare studies. The investigators reported that many studies in HL have used either the REALM or NVS to measure HL, but the REALM focuses more on reading literacy and the NVS focuses more on numeracy literacy (Shigaki et al., 2012). The REALM tool contains a list of 66 medical or healthcare related words that patients are asked to read out loud, with the score being given to match the number of words pronounced correctly. The REALM test takes approximately three to five minutes to administer and score. Test-retest reliability of the REALM has proven as excellent with an alpha Cronbach equaling 0.99 and a $p < .001$. Correlations of the REALM with other popular measures to assess literacy, including the WRAT-R are high, with an r of 0.88.

Ibrahim et al. (2008) conducted a study on coronary heart disease patients that helped validated the REALM tool by comparing it to them, then widely used tool in the United Kingdom, the Basic Skills Agency Initial Assessment Test (BSA) tool, which was used to measure general literacy levels. The study demonstrated that the REALM tool has construct validity for use as a HL screening tool in health-related studies and clinical practice for practitioners seeking to determine HL scores. Results demonstrated validity with an r of 0.70 and a $p < 0.001$. This study concluded that additional studies were necessary to assess the incidence of lower HL within a larger population since the population size was not encompassing of a larger population. Additional studies are needed to identify whether or not there is a relationship between lower HL scores and the poorer population of the United Kingdom (Ibrahim et al., 2008).

Arozullah et al. (2007) conducted a study to demonstrate the validity of the REALM-SF tool. The REALM-SF showed excellent agreement between the REALM-SF and parent REALM instrument. The study revealed that the REALM-SF tool was found to be a valid and reliable measurement tool used to effectively and rapidly measure patient HL scores. The REALM-SF tool demonstrates concurrent criterion validity with its parent tool, the REALM. The REALM-SF tool was developed to provide investigators an opportunity to quickly and accurately facilitate studies in literacy assessment applicable to a variety of clinical scenarios, while reducing the time spent with the patient, thus decreasing risks to the patient (Arozullah et al., 2007). The REALM-SF instrument scores were found to be highly correlated in both development and validation samples, showing $r = 0.94$ and $p <$

0.001, which represent tool validity (Arozullah et al., 2007). Arozullah et al. (2007) concluded that the REALM-SF is considered to be a validated instrument that can be used to assess patient literacy in a variety of diverse clinical study settings.

Synthesis. Although there are many valid and reliable tools available to measure HL, the tools initially considered for use in this DPI project were the WRAT-3, the NVS, and the REALM-SF. The REALM-SF tool was selected for this DPI project as it presents a valid and reliable option to assess HL while allowing for considerations to reduce time spent with the patient, to minimize patient risk. The REALM-SF is a suitable option for all age groups and can be administered and scored within a minute, compared to the three to five minutes required when administering the WRAT-3 or NVS tools. The NVS is primarily utilized to assess numeracy literacy and the WRAT-3 focuses on reading skills, spelling, and mathematics of general literacy, but the REALM-SF tool focuses solely on measuring health literacy as it pertains to healthcare settings. The focus of this DPI project was on health literacy in a healthcare setting and the REALM-SF tool was found to be most appropriate for the setting.

Outcomes and impact. There is a strong association between lower health literacy levels and poor health-related outcomes for patients (Stagliano & Wallace, 2013). MacLeod et al. (2017) conducted a study to estimate the prevalence of inadequate health literacy in older adults, to help identify common characteristics between cohorts when comparing overall health statuses between older adults that are eligible for Medicare programs compared to healthier randomly selected older adults. The impacts of low HL on patient satisfaction were considered as well as the potential need for interventions aimed at a population level targeting older adults with lower HL rates, in particular, those with diminished health statuses. This study surveyed participants within 10 states. Among the 7334 eligible participants in the study, 23% of the ill population was found to have inadequate or low HL compared to 16% of the population sample that was not considered as unhealthy or ill.

Findings of the study revealed common characteristics for lower HL as being common among older males, over age 65 years, with lower education and comorbidities. Findings demonstrated that low HL levels associate with lowering patient satisfaction levels, lower participation in preventative healthcare services, increased use of healthcare services and increased costs for utilizing health services. Discussion points of the study mentioned the concerns surrounding the common prevalence of low to inadequate HL among patients that are making healthcare decisions for themselves that would impact the outcome of their healthcare. Health literacy was found to be an important consideration in successfully managing particular aspects of chronic conditions such as congestive heart failure (CHF) and asthma when compared to other chronic illnesses. Inadequate HL was found to be more common within the older adult population with chronic health conditions, further diminishing health outcome expectations. Recommendations included the potential benefits from additional educational activities or additional care coordination efforts by the healthcare team members (MacLeod et al., 2017).

Mackert et al. (2016) conducted a study, which surveyed 4974 American participants, to define whether HL is associated with patient use of four different HIT tools and applications. Fitness and nutrition applications, exercise and activity tracking apps, and patient portals were the focus of the study. Additionally, the study sought to determine if HL levels were associated with patient perceptions on ease of use and the practicality of the HIT tools. Consideration for patient perceptions related to HIT and privacy, governmental trust, technology companies, and healthcare were explored.

Health literacy levels were measured on all participants. Data collected from participants included patient use of HIT tools and perceived ease of use and the usefulness of the HIT tools. Patients provided demographic information and were also queried about feelings on privacy and trust within healthcare and governmental organizations. Results demonstrated that overall, 15.9%, or 794 out of 4974, showed low HL scores, as measured with the NVS measure of HL tool. The findings revealed that higher HL levels were linked to increased perceived ease of use and usefulness of HIT and lower levels of health literacy correlated to increased perceptions of privacy maintenance by the various HIT tools. Importantly, it was found that participants with lower HL tended to be less trusting of the government and more trusting in healthcare systems. Additional studies were suggested to better understand the implications for using HIT for a preventative nature across large populations.

Bailey et al. (2015) conducted a retrospective cohort study to assess the validity of a predictive model measuring HL. Validity was determined by examining the estimated health literacy levels and comparing them to 30-day hospital readmission rates for patients that had an acute myocardial infarction (AMI). The participant cohort group consisted of 696 patients that were English-speaking adults aged 55 to 74 years old. Variables collected for this study included gender, age, race, education level, income, and chronic condition status.

Three literacy assessments were used to measure HL scores, the REALM, the Test of Functional Health Literacy in Adults (TOFHLA), and the NVS, as all three are proven as valid tools and are considered three of the more commonly used objective measurement tools for HL (Bailey et al., 2015). Results demonstrated that patients who tested as having an above basic HL level showed an 18% lower risk of being readmitted 30 days post discharge and showed a 21% lower incidence rate of 30-day readmission than patients testing as basic or below basic levels of HL. Clinical variables were considered, and after adjusting the analysis to account for demographic variables, the findings revealed that the incidence for readmission was 16% lower for patients with above basic literacy, with a 12% lower risk for readmission. Study conclusions determined that health literacy, when measured as a predictive model, was found to be a significant independent predictor for 30-day readmissions. Recommendations include that HL should be considered to improve patient outcomes in terms of readmission rates.

Synthesis. This subtheme section reviewed studies as they pertain to the outcomes and impact of health literacy levels, in particular as low HL relates to satisfaction and outcomes, patient use of HIT, and readmission rates. Common demographic variables collected in the studies included gender, age, education, and health status. These variables were considered when developing the demographic data collected as part of this DPI project. Findings demonstrated that low health literacy rates do equate to poor health outcomes, lower satisfaction, lower participation in preventative healthcare services, increased costs and increased readmission rates. Higher HL rates correlated to patient use of interventional health-related information technology. The purpose of this quantitative correlational project was to determine to what degree a relationship existed between health literacy scores, measured with the REALM-SF tool, and patient use of the iPET system to view health education modules for telemetry patients at a 225-bed community hospital in the Southwestern United States. This project sought to understand if HL scores have an effect on a patient's propensity to utilize iPET technology for education, which helps to answer gaps as they exist pertaining to the need for additional studies in how to better identify and extract the potential benefits from educational activities by the healthcare team members as they relate to HL and how HL is pertinent to technology as a means of consideration to improve patient outcomes of all patients on a national level.

National considerations. Health literacy concerns have been identified as vital elements of both public and individual health (Cabellos-Garcia et al., 2018). Health literacy impacts patient self-care behaviors, with the emphasis being placed on methods to facilitate and optimize resources to best improve health outcomes (Cabellos-Garcia et al., 2018). Patients with low HL may demonstrate poor health outcomes as well as increased cost utilization when compared to patients with higher HL skills (Cawthon et al., 2014). Investigators that specialize in health literacy consider the impacts that social factors such as poverty levels, educational backgrounds, and geographical locations have on health statuses (Logan et al., 2015). Health literacy rates within the United States are found to be linked to race, ethnicity, income, educational background, and age (Kutner et al., 2006). After adjusting for these variables, HL in itself was found to be an independent risk factor for all-cause mortality rates (Sudore et al., 2006). Smith et al. (2018) found that mortality rates were more than doubled in persons with low literacy when compared to persons with higher literacy rates. Health literacy and related patient outcomes are topics of national concern.

The Institute of Medicine (IOM) recommends integrating health literacy assessment screening into healthcare HIT systems to enable studies measuring the effects of HL on patient outcomes as well as to monitor the best interventions to address HL concerns (IOM, 2004). Healthy People 2020 recognize HL as a key issue within the health and healthcare domain (ODPHP, 2019a). Healthy People 2020 contain several national objectives specific to improving the HL of the United States population. With pertinence to this DPI project are objective HC/HIT-1, to improve the health literacy of the population and objective HC/HIT-2, to increase the number of people that report healthcare practitioners to have satisfactory skills in communication (ODPHP, 2019b). Objective HC/HIT-4 is in continuous development but identifies the goal to increase the percentage of patients whose doctor recommends personalized health information resources, such as HIT, to help the patient manage healthcare options (ODPHP, 2019b). Objective HC/HIT-1.1 identifies the goals about receiving easy-to-understand instructions on how to care for an illness or condition and objective HC/HIT-1.2 aims to increase the number of people that report healthcare practitioners as asking patients to teach back as to how the patient will follow the healthcare instructions provided (ODPHP, 2019b).

With heavy focus on HL as it relates to national considerations and goals, the Health and Human Services (HHS) Health Literacy Workgroup, in conjunction with additional collaborating organizations, established the National Action Plan to Improve Health Literacy (NAPIHL) (Baur, 2011). The NAPIHL is a framework for all healthcare institutions, including nurses, to help identify and address HL barriers that may lead to negative patient outcomes on both the individual and community level (Baur, 2011). The NAPIHL urges healthcare organizations to help identity, select, and implement best healthcare strategies that have the most probable potential to yield positive and measurable improvements in national health literacy rates.

In 2003, the United States conducted the first large-scale national assessment to measure English health literacy (Cutilli & Bennett, 2009). The National Assessment of Adult Literacy (NAAL) was the first national study to contain aspects and indication assessments related to the evaluation of HL in American. The NAAL included health literacy information as a focus to relate to specific health literacy objectives and initiatives within Health People 2020 as well as to establish a baseline assessment of where the American population stood as it relates to reading, understanding, and applying health-related information in the healthcare setting (White, 2008). Increasing attention and emphasis on the importance of HL as it relates to patient outcomes had been established; yet additional studies had only just started linking HL levels to medical errors and overall health disparities when the NAAL was administered throughout the United States (White, 2008). The US Department of Education's National Center for Education Statistics (NCES) (2019) reports that the HL component of the NAAL will be used to establish a baseline for which to measure future progress as it relates to health literacy within the United States.

The results of the study were meant to be descriptive. Interpretation of the results of the NAAL study was meant to reveal relationships between HL and patient demographic and background, not to create causal inferences between the variables collected (Cutilli & Bennett, 2009). More than 19,000 adults were considered eligible participants for this study. Any English-speaking participant over the age of 16 years old was considered an adult for this study (NCES, 2019). Findings of the

NAAL indicate that health literacy is strongly related to general literacy. NAAL results found that approximately 52% of the population had an intermediate level of health literacy, 12% tested as proficient in health literacy, 22% had basic health literacy skills, and 14% had a below basic level of HL (Kutner et al., 2006). There was a combined 36% of the adult population that had a basic or below basic level of HL skills (Kutner et al., 2006).

Characterization of adults with low basic levels of health literacy revealed that these participants might lack basic reading skills and 49% of adults within this category had never attended or had not completed a high school level education (Kutner, 2006). Forty-two percent of participants that tested within the below basic level of health literacy reported having poor overall health and one-third of adults reporting as having fair health, scored within the below basic level of HL. These two findings were statistically higher than adults that reported their health as being good, very good, or excellent. Additional demographic data, in addition to performance data, was collected as it could be relatable to HL including language was spoken before starting school, medical insurance status, age, race, ethnicity, poverty level, prison status, and disability status. Due to the complex nature of connecting all of the relationships between the variables collected, aspects of variable interaction considerations have yet been completely examined (Cutilli & Bennett, 2009).

Results of the NAAL study revealed that participants scoring as intermediate or proficient in health literacy are more likely to seek health information from all sources: print, the internet, radio, television, family, coworkers, and healthcare professionals (Cutilli & Bennett, 2009). Participants that scored as low or below low levels of HL were less likely to utilize a variety of sources to obtain health information and education. Results from the NAAL provide a snapshot of health literacy within the United States. The findings found that the demographics show the following individuals or groups as having a more difficult time understanding healthcare information as it is presented to them: Black or Hispanic, males, persons over the age of 65 years, having less than a high school diploma, living at or below the poverty line, rate overall health as poor, have no insurance or is on Medicare or Medicaid, and do not seek any additional health information from those with higher levels of HL (Kutner et al., 2006). Utilizing the findings from the NAAL study can help healthcare professionals consider which patients are more likely to have lower HL and what is the best method for presenting healthcare information to those patients (Cutilli & Bennett, 2009).

Cawthon et al. (2014) conducted a large academic medical center study that monitored changes made to the nursing assessment of HL and education documentation and how these changes impacted the ease of integration into the electronic health record (EHR). Implementation of new screening forms included the addition of the brief health literacy screen (BHLS) tool as it was used across all of the adult inpatient units, the emergency department, and across three primary care clinics. The study aimed to determine the feasibility and ease of incorporating HL screening into routine clinical assessments while assuring integration into the patient EHR. Additionally, the next steps of the project included the evaluation of how associating HL screening relates to patient care outcomes in both the acute and outpatient settings. The study included monitoring of 55,611 admitted adult inpatients over 18 months and 23,186 adult patients, that over 10 months, made 39, 595 visits to three different primary care clinics.

The findings revealed that nurses in both the inpatient and outpatient settings quickly adapted to using the BHLS tool to measure patient HL (Cawthon et al., 2014). There were noted differences in completion rates between the two settings, with hospital completion rates found to be 90% and overall clinic completions at a significantly lower rate of 67%. Overall, the findings of the study conclude that it is plausible to implement routine brief health literacy screening tools in hospital and clinic settings, yet further studies are necessary to determine the best methods of integrating the health literacy assessments into the patient EHRs. Noted consideration was given to the importance of incorporating HL assessments with patient EHRs. Assuring health literacy information is accessible within the patient EHR will help guide further studies on how lower HL affects patient outcomes and processes of care, as well as focusing studies and projects on how to best distribute educational resources to patients based on individual patient levels of HL.

Yin et al. (2009) conducted a cross-sectional study to assess the health literacy of parents within the United States and to explore the role that HL has in intervening in the health disparities of children. The study aimed to determine if low parental HL levels were correlational between HL and self-reported child health statuses, understanding of medication labels for over the counter (OTC) medication, and proper understanding of food nutrition labels. The sample population was comprised of more than 6100 parents in a generalized form to represent the sample used in the 2003 NAAL survey. Findings from the study concluded that 68.4% of parents were not able to correctly complete health insurance forms by entering names and dates of birth on the form. 28.7% of the parents had basic or below basic HL levels and 65.9% of parents were unable to calculate the annual costs associated with health insurance based upon a family rate. Almost half, or 46.4%, could not perform at least one of two medication-related tasks.

Findings showed that parents with below basic HL levels had increased odds of reporting difficulties with understanding OTC medication labels, at a rate of 3.4 times higher than those parents with HL levels of basic and above (Yin et al., 2009). The study results demonstrate large numbers of parents within the United States have limited or low HL levels and that lower parental health literacy levels reflect the outcomes and issues of illness in children's health statuses. Recommendations stemming from this study include finding methods to reduce the demand for parental HL when parents are caring for their children within the healthcare system. Additional studies are recommended in the areas of how to best design delivery of written forms and education materials, especially as they relate to quantitative literacy skill levels. Studies are needed to determine how health literacy can serve as an indicator to predict health disparities as well as way in which known HL can help to improve the outcomes of known health disparities in children.

Synthesis. Health literacy rates within the United States have been linked to many variables, but HL in itself was found to be an independent risk factor for all-cause mortality rates. Mortality rates were found to double in individuals with low literacy when compared to those with higher literacy levels, emphasizing the importance that HL has on patient outcomes. Health literacy concerns on a national level have led to initiatives to help improve overall HL rates within the United States. Studies have been conducted that indicate there are gaps in the literature in terms of how literacy levels can serve as an indicator to predict health disparities, especially in terms of how technology can best be utilized by nursing to disseminate education resources, in the hopes of improving HL levels that best fit within the national recommendations and guidelines. This DPI project attempts to close the gaps related to patient use of technologies, with nurse oversight, to view education modules and how or if HL can be used as a predictor of such technology use. Utilizing national recommendations as a guideline, nursing must consider how education dissemination can be best utilized on an individual basis and whether technology is the best method for patients with higher literacy levels, overall stressing the need to monitor and assess patient literacy levels on all hospitalized patients.

Nursing considerations. Effective communication techniques between patients and nurses are imperative, as patients and nurses must share information that is mutually understood. As patient advocates, nurses are responsible for delivering care to patients with varying HL levels. Nurses are responsible for delivering healthcare information to patients in a clear and concise manner, yet it is possible that nurses may overestimate patient understanding and comprehension of what is being presented (Christensen, 2016). Patient health outcomes may improve if nurses can recognize barriers to patient HL and understanding. Health literacy levels of patients and families must be considered, and nurses should be prepared to address HL concerns as assessed, but in particular, as they relate to nursing dissemination of patient health education (Eadie, 2014).

Wittenberg et al. (2018) conducted a cross-sectional quantitative survey study to explore oncologic nurse communication challenges with lower literacy patients. The frequency in which oncology nurses assisted with patient literacy needs and any perceived degree of communication difficulties was explored. The perceived comfort level of nurses in dealing and providing HL support was also considered. There were a total of 70 nurse participants in the study. Findings demonstrated that 41% of nurses communicated challenges with low-literacy patient populations that did not speak English as a first language. Nurse recognition of patient literacy levels was based upon the subjective opinion of the nurses and was not measured with a reliable tool that measured or assessed patient HL levels. Nurses that reported patient low literacy levels based concerns upon situations or feelings in which they thought there was a barrier in communication.

There were 36 nurses, or 49% of nurses surveyed, that did not identify patient communication behaviors to indicate low HL (Wittenberg et al., 2018). Continued education to improve HL skills was recommended for nurses at every level. Wittenberg et al. (2018) provided a summary of recommended health literacy tools for nurses that included the use of patient HL assessment tools as well as methods to improve communication strategies, such as by utilizing the teach-back method. Further studies were recommended to rule out subjective biases in future studies as well as to assess the need for more studies involving nurses and how HL support can positively influence patient outcomes.

Matsuoka et al. (2016) conducted a cross-sectional observational study on 227 patients to determine if there were any noted associations between HL and patient self-care behaviors. The study aimed to investigate the relationship between functional and communicative comprehensive HL, critical HL, and self-care behavior in patients with heart failure diagnoses. Over seven months, data was collected willing participant patients diagnosed with heart failure and over the age of 18 years, with the mean age being 67.7 years old. The Heart Failure-Specific Health Literacy Scale was used to assess patient HL levels, and self-care behavior was assessed with a Japanese version of the European Heart Failure Self-Care Behavior Scale (EHFScBS). Patient demographic variable data collected included age, gender, education level, annual income, employment status, and living situations.

Self-care for this study was defined as the level of patient acquisition of knowledge regarding one's current disease process and applying the knowledge in a manner that best suits self-care practices (Matsuoka et al., 2016). Self-care was also described as the decision-making process in which the patient decides the best actions to prevent recurrence of illness, including attending clinical examinations and partaking in the appropriate interventions to remain as healthy as possible. Results demonstrated that patients with low HL levels had poorer knowledge about their health condition and poor self-care behavior when compared to those participants that scored high on the health literacy scale, indicating that critical HL was found to be independently associated with self-care behavior in heart failure patients. The authors concluded that HL was strongly correlated with self-care behavior for patients with heart failure. The authors identified an implication for practice as utilizing the findings to change the methods in which patients with heart failure are educated. Teach-back methods are strongly advised as well as delivering education in more than one method besides written material.

Griffey et al. (2015) performed a randomized, controlled study of 408 adult patients with low HL, to assess the effectiveness of teach-back versus standard discharge instructions in patients discharged from the emergency department. The study examined whether teach-back improved comprehension and perceived comprehension of discharge instructions provided to patients as well as satisfaction among patients with limited or low HL levels. The data was collected over an approximate 2-month period and HL levels were measured with the Rapid Estimate of Adult Literacy in Medicine-Revised (REALM-R). Patients that scored less than a six on the REALM-R were considered as having low HL and eligible for participation. Exclusion criteria included patients unable to speak, non-English speaking, mentally handicapped, and patients visiting the emergency department because of psychiatric, clinical intoxication, or sexual assault. Patients were provided the REALM-R tool and then randomly selected to receive teach-back discharge or standard discharge instructions based upon whether the last digit in the medical record number was an odd or even number.

Chi-square tests were used to examine the demographic differences between the two groups and bivariate associations were conducted between the teach-back versus standard discharge group and the study outcomes of comprehension, perceived comprehension, and satisfaction groups (Griffey et al., 2015). Multivariable ordinal logistic regression models were utilized to examine the effects of one study group with the outcome variables, with adjustments being made for racial demographic data. Statistical significance was consistent, with a p-value of <0.05. Notations regarding race were notes as patients who received teach-back had significantly higher comprehension results compared with patients who received standard discharge instructions.

Discussion notes indicate that this study was the first to explore the use of teach-back in the ED, as no prior randomized controlled studies examined the effectiveness of using teach-back methods to improve comprehension of discharge education in the emergency department among patients with known low HL levels (Griffey et al., 2015). Results demonstrated that patients that received teach-back instructions had higher compensation of post-discharge care, specifically in terms of post-discharge medication, self-care instructions, and follow-up instructions. There was no change in patient satisfaction or perceived comprehension of discharge care. The study conclusions support the effectiveness of using teach-back as an effective measure of understanding, yet additional studies are recommended to test the feasibility of using teach-back for routine use, especially pertaining to the impacts on longer term outcomes.

Synthesis. Effective communication between nurse and patient is imperative; especially as it pertains to providing patient education and promoting positive patient self-care behaviors since patient HL levels can impede optimal communication or receptive understanding of provided education. When providing education to patients, nurses should not assume the patient understands the directions or education; rather they should consider the capacity for patient understanding or patient HL status of each patient. The teach-back method can be utilized by nurses to assure patients understand the information presented to them and to assess any barriers that may exist with comprehension. Gaps in the literature demonstrate the need for further studies in teach-back techniques, especially in how education is presented to patients with chronic disease statuses, such as heart failure. This DPI project assessed HL levels on telemetry patients before educating patients on the use the iPET as an available means to view educational videos. Analysis of understanding was conducted through the teach-back method to assure understanding of the information presented, allowing the focus to remain on the dependent variable of HL levels, as a means to determine the patient propensity to utilize interactive patient engagement technology for patient education.

PATIENT EDUCATION

Patient education is an integral factor in improving patient satisfaction, healthcare quality, and cost (Latimer, 2018). Integrating HIT and patient education techniques promotes and encourages patients to take an active role in their own healthcare decisions, improve understanding and adherence to care plans, and fosters improved communication with patients and healthcare clinicians (Latimer, 2018). The delivery of patient education falls heavily on nurses, yet much of the profession is lacking in the knowledge and expertise of assessing patient HL levels as they relate to delivering effective patient education (Kennard, 2016). Increasing adaptability of digital health-related applications and the use of other innovative HIT enhances patient outcomes when delivering personalized education to patients on the individual patient level (Latimer, 2018). Interventions found to help improve patient self-care led to improvements in patient self-efficacy (Paterick et al., 2017). Patient education is considered a key aspect of nursing as it fosters patient-nurse communication, promotes patient involvement and shared decision making, assist patients in making decisions based off of provider recommendations, and engages patients to partake in self-care decisions involving their care (Cassano, 2019).

Teach-back. The delivery of education, through healthcare encounters, should promote patient engagement and discussion (Wolf & Bailey, 2009). To confirm that patients have understood the information and education provided to them about medical conditions, medications, treatments, and care plans, nurses can use the teach-back method (Wolf & Bailey, 2009). Through teach back intervention, nurses can assess and reassess educational needs on an individual patient level, to assure that full comprehension of technology explanation has occurred (Wilson et al., 2012). The teach-back method can be utilized as a means to improve and foster communication between patients and healthcare workers. Not only will using the teach-back method help promote discussion between the patient and nurse, but can also help prevent potential errors or actions that may result because of patient misunderstandings with education materials presented to them (Wolf & Bailey, 2009). When utilizing the teach-back method, patients may be asked to confirm their understanding of the education material by repeating back, in their verbiage, what their understanding is of the material is or may be asked questions that pinpoint specific information, such as by asking the patient what they found to be the most important aspect of the learning (Bullen & Young, 2016). In all regards, the teach-back method is an effective means to improve patient-provider or patient-nurse communication (Wolf & Bailey, 2009). I patient education techniques are not proving effective, patient HL should be considered.

Bullen and Young (2016) conducted a case study regarding the various self-care behaviors that are necessary for diabetic patients to avoid foot ulcerations. The study explained that all patients were provided verbal and written education, describing the best methods to avoid foot ulcers, at every visit to reinforce patient intervention and promote positive self-care behaviors. The study sought to determine whether HL status should be considered in the cases in which patients continued to develop foot ulcers, despite the methods taken to improve the patient's knowledge of proper self-care actions and behaviors necessary to avoid the development of ulcers. The case study pinpoints an example of where the patient education had failed to prevent a foot ulcer in a patient with diabetes and peripheral vascular disease. Patient HL levels were screened, and the teach-back method was utilized.

The patient had received both verbal and written materials directed at how to prevent diabetic foot ulcers, yet did develop additional foot ulcers after this education (Bullen & Young, 2016). Written patient education materials provided to the patient described recommendations against using over-the-counter corn remedies and to contact the local foot clinic in the event that an ulcer did develop. The patient neglected to follow either of these advised instructions, despite having been seen in the clinic on several prior occasions, with this educational information being reinforced each time. Patient HL, to determine if there was a barrier to the ability for the patient to understand the directions, was assessed with the Single Item Literacy Screener (SILS) tool. Conclusions of the study found that assessing HL levels before educational interventions may help nurses better understand the best avenues to provide educational materials to patients and that the teach-back method would be useful as a means to confirm whether the patient fully understood the material being presented, especially as it pertains to patient self-care behaviors.

Wilson et al. (2012) conducted a study to assess maternal HL of pregnant women in Jamaica, to assess their understanding of the benefits, risks, and safety of two vaccines after using the teach-back method as part of the educational intervention. This study reiterated the global concerns regarding low HL levels in women, as women comprise nearly two-thirds of the world's estimated 960 million illiterate adults. Several demographic variables were collected as data in the study from the 34 eligible participants, which included patient age, race, health insurance, spoken language, educational background, ethnicity, and income. HL scores were measured with the REALM tool. The teach-back method was utilized to assure understanding and retention of educational information provided to the participants.

Results of the study demonstrated an average HL level for the participants fell within the low literacy levels (Wilson et al., 2012). The study also demonstrated that the teach-back method proved to be effective for participants with higher literacy levels; there were no statistically significant gains for women with lower literacy levels. Conclusions from the study revealed the importance for nursing to assess HL levels on patients as well as have an awareness or knowledge of what literacy levels particular education material is meant to target. Continued efforts are necessary to form collaborations between healthcare professionals and nursing in order to determine the best innovative methods to benefit patients with lower literacy levels.

Wilson et al. (2008) conducted a study, guided by Orem's SCDNT, to assess the relationship between maternal HL and the ability to understand and verbalize information about childhood immunizations. The study focused on communication, particularly with an emphasis on patients that have low literacy skills. Because there are gaps in the literature about a lack of existing studies that focus on the patient's ability to communicate health information given to them by healthcare professionals, the PI determined the study important in purpose. There were a total of 30 participant mothers, split into two groups based upon whether they had only one child or more than one child. Orem's SCDNT was used as the conceptual framework in this study. Based on Orem's theory, basic capabilities to perform foundational skills such as reading, writing, verbalization, counting, and reasoning are all necessary components to the individual's ability to perform self-care (Wilson et al., 2008).

The design type used for this study was a mixed quantitative and qualitative design. Demographic data collected included age, education level, insurance, family structure, and method of transportation to the clinics (Wilson et al., 2008). The REALM was used to assess HL statuses and quantitative collection of teach-back responses were calculated using quantitative analysis. Teach-back responses were assessed based upon whether the patient responded correctly on all answers, if they were partially correct, or had incorrect answers. Chi-square tests were conducted to associate the number of children with the patient's ability to communicate immunization benefits, risks, and the safety of the vaccines. Fisher's Exact Test was used to determine the statistical significant differences between groups regarding the teach-back responses. There were limitations in the study due to small sample sizes, which also removed the generalizability of this study to a more general population.

Results demonstrated a lack of statistical significance between the ability to communicate correct teach-back responses based upon the number of children the mother had (Wilson et al., 2008). Patients with lower literacy skills had more partially correct or incorrect responses than those with higher literacy scores. There were inconsistencies noted with the mother's ability to communicate critical information via teach-back, demonstrating the need for further studies to assess the best methods to deliver immunization information to patients, as the manner in which education is presented to patients, based upon literacy scores, is pertinent and unless effective communication strategies are utilized, there will be limited successes when attempting to increase HL (Wilson et al., 2008).

Synthesis. Barriers in a patient's ability to read, write, count, reason, or communicate can impact their ability to properly perform self-care behaviors that may be taught to them by nursing staff during educational interventions. When patient education techniques are not proving to be effective or when barriers are identified, HL levels should be considered. Patients may present with low health literacy or cannot understand the education being provided, therefore unable to properly follow the recommended self-care behaviors that will promote the most optimal outcomes. Literacy levels may impact the effectiveness of teaching as well as the patient's ability to verbalize back to the nurse what was discussed and learned. How education is presented should be tailored to their HL level, to assure patients are presented with education in the manner that best fits their ability to understand it. This DPI project measured HL levels on all participants as well as utilized teach-back techniques, as a means to fill gaps in the literature surrounding the lack of studies as they pertain to health literacy levels and their effect on the use of self-care technological interventions such as the iPET.

HIT

HHS (2019) defines HIT as the exchange of health data within an electronic setting. To assure patient health information (PHI) remains confidential and protected, privacy and security concerning HIT is of key concern and priority. Increased use of HIT tools within the healthcare environment will improve the quality of healthcare delivered, decreasing the number of medically related errors, reduce healthcare-associated costs, and expand access to affordable healthcare for Americans (HHS, 2019). Integrating HIT within the nursing profession has been beneficial for both nursing and patient outcomes, especially as technologies improve and better methods to improve patient care are discovered (Cassano, 2019). Of particular importance is the emphasis placed on patient education and patient engagement with HIT (Cassano, 2019). Ongoing studies are imperative to continue to understand the benefits that technology can have upon patient experiences (Werder, 2015).

The Office of the National Coordinator for Health IT (ONC) is responsible for overseeing the advancement of connectivity and operations involving HIT within the

United States. ONC's jurisdiction is the oversight of patient education and patient engagement about HIT. Proper education and engagement techniques provide patients with information that is easily accessible, direct, and clear for understanding (ONC, 2018). Patient education and patient engagement are crucial aspects of HIT considerations. Studies have yielded national consideration regarding HIT and patient outcomes (Bowles, Dykes, & Demiris, 2015). National policies, such as the Health Information Technology for Economic and Clinical Health (HITECH) Act have been implemented to improve patient safety and improve the quality and efficiency of delivered healthcare (Bowles et al., 2015).

Information technology within the healthcare arena can play an important role in improving a patient's healthcare understanding and experience as a whole (Werder, 2015). Interventions delivered via healthcare technology devices can improve patient understanding of information and instructions being provided and promote patient health literacy (Jacobs, 2015). There are many technologies available to help enhance patient literacy; healthcare clinicians must expand their use of technologies to target conditional and patient-centered technologies (Jacobs, 2015).

As technology in healthcare advances, it is imperative that nurses find the right balance while utilizing technology in the healthcare setting and providing quality patient care. Patient care has become a key focus about the growth of new ideas and concepts involving healthcare technologies (Cassano, 2015). Utilization of HIT in nursing practice can assure delivery of precise, easily accessible, and actionable information targeted directly to patients, to allow open communication between patients and healthcare clinicians (Huston, 2013). Current healthcare trends focus on patient care as it relates to clinical applications and technologies which emphasize communication between healthcare team members and patients. Patient education delivery through the use of bedside technology devices has shown that proper understanding and knowledge of these devices can reduce re-admission rates, improve healing times, decrease mental discomforts, and yield overall improved patient outcomes about disease processes (Cassano, 2015). Nursing interventions tailored to the delivery of patient education through technology, when carried out effectively, can improve patient self-care and coping skills (Cassano, 2015).

Patient engagement. Patient engagement focuses on the attainment of patient participation and involvement in self-care practices and behaviors, under the pretense that patients will take an active interest and role in the outcomes of their illness and disease processes. Patient engagement focuses on the relationship between healthcare clinicians and patients, as they work in conjunction to promote and support patient involvement in their own self-care and healthcare choices (Carman et al., 2013). Carman et al. (2013) defines patient and family engagement as the process for both patients and families, as they work in active partnership with healthcare clinicians, at varying levels of healthcare organizations, including the governmental level, to improve health outcomes and healthcare practices for consumers and American citizens. The Health Information Management Systems Society (HIMSS) defines patient engagement as the process of clinicians and patients working together to improve health (2019). HIMSS (2019) identifies patient and family engagement opportunities when patients partake in available hits, such as patient health portals, secure health messaging, social media, and emerging health-related technologies.

Assessing patient engagement can be imperative as a means to enhance patient health and reduce healthcare-associated costs (Nunlist, Blumberg, Uiterwyk & Apgar, 2016). Patients that are engaged and involved in their healthcare have better health outcomes, report positive healthcare experiences, are less likely to utilize healthcare services, and cost less than patients that are not engaged (Wasson & Coleman, 2014). Patient engagement and participation in self-care behaviors can be affected by extrinsic factors such as health status, socioeconomic stresses, quality of healthcare. Active patient engagement is associated with improved patient outcomes and lower use of healthcare services (Nunlist et al., 2016). Measuring patient health confidence allows practitioners to determine patient engagement, which allows for proper interventions to yield improved patient outcomes (Nunlist et al., 2016).

Nunlist et al. (2016) conducted a study of 287 patients to determine if patient health confidence levels affected patient health outcomes and influenced healthcare related costs. Five different physicians and four nurse practitioners and physician assistants measured health confidence levels on patients in a family practice clinic over one year. To calculate health confidence levels, patients were asked to rate the level in which they felt confident they could control and manage most of their health issues. Patients responded with a numerical answer on a scale ranging from zero to ten, with zero having no confidence and ten being extremely confident. Results of the study determined that patients with high or improved health confidence scores led to lower use of hospital care and thus a decrease in costs associated with care. Recommendations from the study included routine assessment of health confidence levels for all patients, to better identify and focus on patients with lower health confidence or lower patient engagement, as well as provide intensive interventions to patients that score lower on the scale, to enhance and boost confidence and promote patient engagement in care.

HIT helps create a bridge for engaging patients and connecting patients to their healthcare team, yet it can be difficult for healthcare team members to measure the effectiveness of patient engagement in connection with patient use of HIT (Solomon, 2014). Solomon (2014) found discrepancies in what is considered a patient engagement indicator. Variations in what patient engagement indicators support the need for a framework that would guide the range and usefulness of HIT interventions that help engage patients (Solomon, 2014). Solomon proposed a health information technology for patient engagement effectiveness (HIT-PE2) model to inform organizations of their personal HIT strategies while evaluating the effectiveness of patient engagement applications. The model seeks to expand beyond the measurement of patient engagement technologies and seeks to create a universal paradigm for measuring patient engagement through technologies. The HIT-PE2 model encompasses the concepts of fostering clinician and patient collaboration in care while emphasizing the importance of patient self-management.

The HIT-PE2 model is based on three main components: system use, patient experience, and patient activation (Solomon, 2014). System use indicators are determined by patient usage of the technology available. Patient experience evaluations are conducted by inquiring about patient satisfaction with the application, perceived usefulness and relevance, and the possibility of recommending the system to others. Patient activation is essentially another term for patient engagement, as highly activated patients are highly engaged patients. A highly activated patient can be defined as a patient engaged in the decisions regarding their healthcare through partaking in the activities and actions provided through interventions with healthcare team members. Additional determinants of activated patients can be measured through the patient's collaboration efforts with providers and nurses, by the patient's actively seeking out knowledge and education on disease processes, and when patients face challenges with confidence as they encounter barriers to care. Solomon (2014) discusses the necessity for more studies to determine the best methods that HIT can help facilitate engagement for patients throughout the United States.

The last known national health literacy survey, conducted in 2003, revealed that only 11% of Americans are HL proficient enough to complete necessary tasks that would allow successful navigation through a healthcare system, such as successfully carrying out instructions and education provided to them during healthcare visits (Kutner et al., 2006). Because there is a necessary need to improve HL rates in America, Koh et al. (2013) proposed the Health Literate Care Model (HLCM), based on the premise that all healthcare providers must approach patients with the supposition that all patients are at risk for not understanding important education and information provided to them, which would inhibit improvements in their health statuses and health outcomes. The proposed HLCM potentially creates an integrated organizational approach to foster patient engagement.

Use of the proposed model would focus on HL and patient engagement while addressing performance goals that address health literacy discrepancies and providing organizational-wide communication training and HL assessment skills (Koh et al., 2013). The HLCM proposes utilizing teach-back techniques during every patient interaction while providing self-management techniques while using plain language and health literacy-focused approach. Patient decision support through the HLCM focuses on providing the patient self-paced, interactive patient decision aids that allow clinicians to engage in shared decision-making discussions with patients. Clinical informatics support under the HLCM would include reminders to nursing staff to conduct health literacy-related tasks. Conclusively, the HLCM would represent a practical framework for healthcare organizations to utilize to consider all patients' HL concerns in a proactive manner by allowing patients to understand the healthcare options, best utilize resources, improve wellness through prevention, and enhance relationships between patients and members of the healthcare team.

Technology is transforming healthcare and the manner in which nursing care is delivered to patients. Technology-enabled healthcare coordination allows nurses to engage with patients over longer periods, as nurses can utilize technology to create patient care plans from before admission to discharge (Hull, 2015). Additionally, nurses can use HIT to delivery education, use surveying tools, assess patients, and use communicative functionality to deliver healthcare information to patients, opening a more dynamic form of communication between patients and nurses in follow up (Hull, 2015). Providing technology to patients in healthcare allows patients to recognize gaps in their care plan, identify potential barriers to maintaining adherence to provider orders, assess and recognize areas of misunderstanding, and better self-monitor health conditions (Danis et al., 2014). Integrating inclusive patient technology into nurse workflows could result in improved adherence, reductions in costs related to care, delivery of targeted, accurate information, and over improve the quality of patient care delivered (Danis et al., 2014).

Zan et al. (2015) conducted a study on patient engagement to evaluate the use and practicality of using the iGetBetter system to promote patient self-management in patients with heart failure. The iGetBetter system is a web and telephone based remote monitoring program to track heart failure symptoms, empowering and allowing patients to take advantage of mobile technologies to monitor their health outside of the acute care facility setting. The study, conducted over 90 days, included 20 adult ambulatory patients with heart failure. Patients used the iGetBetter interventional system to record their weight, blood pressure, and heart rate every morning using a special Bluetooth weight scale and self-inflating blood pressure cuff, both connected to an iPad mini tablet with access to the internet. Data was loaded to an internet site, and data was accessible by the patient via that site.

Patient outcomes assessed included patient satisfaction with the device, patient engagement with the intervention, heart failure-related quality of life, and the utilization of hospital resources (Zan et al., 2015). Results reflect that 95% of participants reported feeling more connected with their healthcare clinicians as well as feeling confident in their self-care behaviors and activities. Heart-failure quality of life scores improved from the baseline, but the results were not found to be statistically significant. About 90% of patients declared feeling better prepared and open to communication with providers regarding their health statuses. Engagement was measured by the number of times a week that the patient used the devices and results measured that 80% had weekly over all weekly engagement with the device.

All participants reported finding the devices that measure weight and blood pressure as easy to use and likable (Zan et al., 2015). It was noted that intervention participants demonstrated shorter than the average length of stays when hospitalized, but there were no noted significant differences observed in this aspect between the control groups and participation groups. Conclusions to the study supported the practicality and feasibility of using a low-demand remote monitoring intervention program for ambulatory patients with heart failure.

Synthesis. Patient engagement, or the level in which patients actively participate and partake in self-care behaviors that affect their health outcomes, can affect patient health outcomes. HIT is one means of promoting patient engagement and patient involvement in healthcare decisions, yet more studies are needed to identify the best methods of technology necessary to help engage patients. Studies focusing on patient health literacy and its effect on patient engagement have been conducted as well as the literature surrounding frameworks that integrate health literacy, teach-back methods, and patient engagement. Recommendations stemming from these proposed frameworks include proposals to measure baseline health literacy levels on all patients admitted to a hospital, to assess their health literacy, to tailor patient interventions to each patient accordingly. Literature shows positive outcomes surrounding patient telehealth technologies, yet gaps in the literature exist relating to how HL scores may impact patient use of self-care interactive technology, such as the iPET as well as how self-care through engagement may impact use of technologies such as the iPET. In this DPI project, HL levels were assessed, and patient use of the iPET was monitored, since the iPET system is self-controlled by the patient, using it to receive health education, can be classified as a self-care behavior.

IPET

HIT systems, aimed at increasing patient engagement to improve patient outcomes, have been becoming increasingly more popular in healthcare (Prey et al., 2014). Nursing is consistently adapting to new technologies in practice as simple as the use of pumps and monitoring electronic specialty equipment to the integration of electronic documentation through EHRs. Early studies that focus on patient-centered HIT have revealed positive outcomes involving increased patient engagement, improved communication, and encouraged contribution to patient self-care behaviors (Dalal et al., 2016).

Interactive Patient Engagement Technology (iPET) systems are defined as electronic systems, used by patients and families, in a hospital or outpatient environment, that help promote patient inclusion and patient participation in self-care techniques (Gee & Patmon, 2016). iPET systems can be used to deliver messages and education videos to patients at home to prepare patients for upcoming medical interventions, such as a procedure or surgery or iPET systems can be provided to patients while hospitalized, through bedside tablets or integrated functionality in the television-based system remote controls (Gee & Patmon, 2016). iPET options for patients at the bedside, in the inpatient setting, include options for patients to watch on-demand Hollywood films, listen to music, view meditation channels, or deliver patient-specific prescribed education material directly to the tablet or television in the patient's own hospital room (Gee & Patmon, 2016).

One of the goals of the iPET system is to increase patient engagement through the use of technology (Patmon et al., 2016). Nursing integration of iPET systems into workflow practice has been especially helpful in terms of providing patient education through the iPET system, as nursing can educate the patient on use and functionality of how to view the prescribed health videos, allowing patient viewing autonomy (Gee & Patmon, 2016). This method of delivering educational material can enhance communication between patient and nurse as the patients can provide teach-back methods to nurses after viewing education modules, allowing nurses to assess any additional learning needs of the patient (Gee & Patmon, 2016).

Because patient engagement is a newer concept within healthcare, most literature and studies pertaining to the outcomes related to patient engagement technology, within an inpatient setting, is derived from qualitative methods, indicating that additional studies are necessary to fill gaps related to quantitative study findings regarding patient engagement as it relates to HIT (Prey et al., 2015). Both healthcare providers and nurses must remain up to date on the latest concepts and technologies, to discover the best methods for engaging patients and directing patients towards self-care behaviors that will improve patient outcomes. Within the confines of current practices and integration of HIT into healthcare, informed patients will not be the norm of care, and it is up to healthcare clinicians to discover, shape, and foster patients' knowledge through the delivery of interventions via HIT (Henwood et al., 2003).

Interventional aspects. Patmon et al. (2016) conducted a descriptive qualitative study to collect the opinion and perceptions of nurses that were integrating the iPET system into daily nursing patient-care workflows. This study aimed to identify barriers that may affect the nursing promotion of the iPET as well as to identify factors for which nurses may promote patient use of the iPET, especially with consideration of integrating the iPET into daily nursing workflows. There were 38 nurses interviewed, from two different hospitals in the western United States. Nurses interviewed included both clinical staff nurses as well as nurses in a leadership role. Nurses were interviewed as well as observed in practice. Results from the study demonstrated that the overall perception from nurses was that the iPET would be beneficial in the enhancement of patient care, as the iPET is integrated into nursing workflows.

Of the options available for patient use with the iPET, early nurse perceptions were found to favor the personal entertainment functionality, which included the ability for patients to play interactive games as well as that of listening to music and watching television. At the time of this study, full integration and full functionality of the iPET was not complete, leaving some functionality in question by nursing staff. For example, nurses were particularly interested in the full benefits of the educational offerings of the iPET system. In the areas in which the educational options were fully implemented, nurses had favorable opinions on the iPET as a means to deliver education modules through the delivery of individualized and patient-specific provider prescribed videos that review pertinent patient education regarding illness and disease processes. Nursing had favorable reviews on educational iPET functionality, indicating the educational intervention would change slightly in that they would not be delivering the initial education to patients first hand, rather focus on intervening through follow up using a teach-back methodology to assure proper patient understanding of the video module.

Discussion notes from the study identify the overall consensus that nurses did perceive the iPET system as one that could enhance patient engagement and could positively impact clinical practice and workflows. Acute care facilities could benefit and enhance clinical nursing practice through iPET uses such as distractions, anxiety reduction, and patient education. Recommendations were tailored to organizations seeking to implement the iPET as part of their routine patient care and discussed assuring adequate training be conducted on nursing staff, with emphasis on allowing adequate time for training, while stressing that training should be specific to how nurses can use the technology to enhance clinical practice and workflows. Findings from the study emphasize the integral importance that nursing has on the patient successful use of the iPET. Nurses are the keys to assuring patient utilization of the iPET systems and to assure the full benefit and functionality of the iPET is taught to patients, as proper education on the instructions for use and functionality are crucial.

Dalal et al. (2016) implemented a web-based, patient-centered toolkit to engage patients and caregivers in their plan of care while hospitalized through the facilitation of education and emphasis on patient and provider communication techniques. Patient participants included 239 hospitalized patients on either a medical intensive care unit or an oncology unit. The purpose of the Dalal et al. (2016) study was to determine how patients can utilize HIT tools to actively participate in their care, while utilizing patient engagement as a foundation to enhance communication with patients and healthcare clinicians, promote positive self-care behavioral changes, and improve the understanding and adherence of instructions provided regarding patient self-care. The goal was to determine what efforts may result in measurable favorable outcomes, lower costs, and improvements in self-care management.

Dalal et al. (2016) designed and developed a patient-centered toolkit (PCTK) to provider patients and caregivers the necessary means and HIT tools to participate in their care plan during hospitalization via electronic means. Patients that were excluded from participation included any patient that was intubated, had an altered mental status, did not speak English, or was visually impaired to the point where they could not see the interactive technology devices. Patients were provided hospital-issued iPads and asked to access the PCTK, update patient goals, view scheduled testing, access and navigate available educational content and message members of the care team directly. Teach-back sessions were conducted to assure patient understanding was achieved.

The findings revealed that more patients on the non-critical oncology unit were willing participants when compared to the patients in the intensive care unit. Patients that did enroll using the PCTK used the device to establish healthcare goals, view test results, and medication, and identify members of the care team. Educational content usage was found to be heavily utilized for reviewing patient medication and test results, but education based on the patient problem or illness was rarely utilized. Recommendations for further studies included examining how clinical outcomes could be impacted by PCTK technology, how PCTK could improve patient self-care, improvement of care plan coordination, ways PCTK could prevent harm and promote safety, and ways in which PCTK could improve patient satisfaction.

White et al. (2013) conducted a prospective cohort study to determine if heart failure patients educated with the teach-back method would retain self-care educational information and whether the teach-back was associated with a decreased rate of hospital readmissions. Data was collected for 276 patients over the age of 65 years over 13 months. Patient participants were hospitalized with a heart failure diagnosis. Nursing used the teach-back method to educate and evaluate the patient understanding of information and directions given. Patients correctly responded to 75% of self-care teach back questions at a rate of approximately 85% of the time while hospitalized and 77% of the time when questioned over the telephone. Results demonstrated that patients who responded to teach back questions correctly while either in the hospital or over the phone, yielded non-significant reduction findings in all-cause hospital readmission rates at 30 days. In contrast, significant findings were found in patients who did have readmissions to the hospital with heart failure.

Conclusions noted from this study identify teach-back as an effective method to both educate and assess patient learning (White et al., 2013). The patients that nursing spent a long time with demonstrated significantly higher retention rates than patients that nurses spent less time with on education. Recommendations for future studies identified randomized studies to compare readmission rates with teach-back education techniques to further compare the effectiveness of teach-back methods.

Synthesis. An iPET system is a form of education delivery and self-directed bedside technology which allows patients to engage in their healthcare choices while taking some control in their health education by watching provider prescribed videos that pertain to the patient's illness or health status. Additional uses of the iPET include utilizing distraction techniques through relaxation and meditation channels and entertainment purposes, such as watching films or listening to music. Nurse perceptions investigated during early integrations of the iPET highlighted anticipation about utilizing the iPET as an educational intervention, with follow up assessments occurring through teach-back that fosters discussion and communication. Early studies on the use of interactive technologies to engage patients through education have revealed a lack of patient interest in using the technologies to educate themselves on their patient illness or health concern. This leaves gaps in the literature regarding the ways in which education interventions through interactive technology can improve outcomes as well as gaps in the literature regarding patient usage of the iPET itself since existing studies highlight nurse perceptions and not patient perceptions. There was no literature found that links health literacy and patient use of the iPET system, thus helping the development of this DPI project, as the PI attempts to fill these gaps by reviewing patient engagement and use of the iPET for education as it relates to patient HL.

SUMMARY

Highly applicable to most nursing settings, the SCDTN focuses on the communication between patients and nurses, with an emphasis on engaging patients to participate in their care through self-care behaviors (Orem & Taylor, 2011). Self-care behaviors are necessary to satisfy ongoing self-care needs that promote positive outcomes and overall healthy well-being (Villarruel et al., 2001). Internal and external factors may prohibit a patient from completing self-care behaviors that promote improved health and positive outcomes (Villarruel et al., 2001). A lack of comprehension or any issues with decision-making abilities or judgments are considered barriers to one's ability to conduct necessary self-care behaviors (Orem, 2001). Nursing must remain vigilant and assure they can identify and address any barriers to patient self-care, so that the barriers can be addressed, allowing patients to fully comprehend the information being provided to them about their healthcare (Orem, 2001).

Health literacy impacts patient self-care behaviors, with the emphasis being placed on methods to facilitate and optimize resources to best improve health outcomes (Cabellos-Garcia et al., 2018). Patient HL is the capacity to obtain, process, and comprehend basic health information or services presented to them so that they can make informed decisions about their health decisions (NASEM, 2015). When considering a patient's HL, the cognitive, social, and navigational skills of the patient must be considered (Lambert & Keogh, 2014). Nurse assessment of patient understanding and comprehension can be accomplished through the teach-back method (Badaczewski et al., 2017). This is a significant consideration as improving HL, and patient communication, allows patients to understand learning material regarding their illness better (ODPHP, 2017c). Additionally, literature has pointed healthcare practitioners and nurses in the direction of measuring patient health literacy, especially as a means to identify and predict which patients may have barriers to learning, which may inhibit improved patient outcomes or improvements in health status (Bailey et al., 2015). Patients with low health literacy may demonstrate poor outcomes when compared to patients with higher health literacy (Cawthon et al., 2014).

Health literacy concerns have become a national priority, as HL has become a crucial element to health outcomes in both individual and population health (Cabellos-Garcia et al., 2018). As of 2003, only 12% of the United States population is considered to be proficient in HL, leaving most of the nation with some deficit of properly understanding healthcare information or how to properly utilize healthcare services (Kutner et al., 2006). In order to address these concerns, objectives, and recommendations to identify and address health literacy concerns have been established through national action plans and addressed in national health improvement initiatives such as Healthy People 2020 (White, 2008). Healthcare systems, providers, and nurses play a vital role in improving HL, as they work in conjunction with patients to identify lower HL levels and analyze patient understanding of healthcare education materials (HHS, 2008).

Health literacy can be measured by a variety of different valid and reliable tools. The REALM-SF tool was found to be most applicable for use in this DPI project, as it was found to be both a valid and reliable tool which can be quickly administered and scored in less than one minute (Arozullah et al., 2007). Decreasing the total time spent with the patient minimizes patient risk (Arozullah et al., 2007). The REALM-SF was found to be a suitable option for all age groups (Alqudah et al., 2014), making it highly applicable to this DPI project where patient participants covered patients ranging from their twenties to their eighties. Nurse assessment of HL on all patients can help improve patient outcomes

Nurses are responsible to deliver healthcare information to patients in a clear and concise manner, yet it is possible that nurses may overestimate patient understanding and comprehension of what is being presented (Christensen, 2016). All patients are at risk of misunderstanding or lacking comprehension of important educational materials presented to them (Koh et al., 2013). Health literacy levels of all patients and families must be considered (Eadie, 2014). Nurses should be prepared to address HL concerns, but in particular, as they relate to nursing dissemination of patient health education (Eadie, 2014). It is imperative to not only recognize deficits in understanding but to use health literacy in a manner as to help predict which patients are at risk (Bailey et al., 2015). Learning the HL status of all patients would allow nursing to tailor education interventions to patients on an individual basis (Danis et al., 2014). Examples such as using interactive HIT devices or systems, such as the iPET, may prove beneficial for some patients with lower HL or barriers with understanding written material. Nurses proficient in HIT can help patients connect electronically to education modules that will help promote improved healthcare related behaviors and improve positive outcomes post hospitalization (Huston, 2013).

Technology is transforming healthcare and how nursing care is delivered to patients. Integrating healthcare related technologies in healthcare plans allows nurses to enhance communication through follow up discussions and teach-back sessions after the patient views videos through the iPET. Additionally, nurses can use HIT to delivery education, use surveying tools, assess patients, and use communicative functionality to deliver healthcare information to patients, opening a more dynamic form of communication between patients and nurses in follow up (Hull, 2015). Providing technology to patients in healthcare allows patients to recognize gaps in their care plan, identify potential barriers to maintaining adherence to provider orders, assess and recognize areas of misunderstanding, and better self-monitor health conditions (Danis et al., 2014). Integrating patient inclusive technology into nurse workflows could result in improved adherence, reductions in costs related to care, delivery of targeted, accurate information, and over improve the quality of patient care delivered (Danis et al., 2014).

Prey et al. (2013) discuss various interactive patient engagement technology devices currently found in the inpatient setting, yet it is noted specifically that further studies are needed, as gaps exist about patient engagement and participation with interactive patient devices in an acute setting (Prey et al., 2013). Additional methodological studies and more practical studies relating to inpatient engagement are needed to explore the best methods to improve patient outcomes (Prey et al., 2013). Existing gaps in the literature form a foundation of significance to guide this project, as in terms of related HL scores with particular HIT delivery through the iPET. It was not known if health literacy scores, measured with the REALM-SF tool, correlated to adult telemetry inpatient use of the iPET to view health education modules when compared to a similar group that did not use the iPET, after both groups of patients were provided the same instructions on functionality and use of the iPET system.

Chapter 3 will detail the quantitative methodology for the DPI project. Chapter 3 will expand upon the project methodology, project design, population and sample selection, tools used for this project, validity, reliability, data collection procedures, data analysis procedures, ethical considerations, and project limitations. Chapter 3 documents how the project was conducted with details that allow for replication of the project.

CHAPTER 3: Methodology

Healthcare systems, providers, and nurses play a vital role in improving health literacy, as these teams work in conjunction with patients to identify low HL levels and analyze patient levels of understanding of the healthcare education materials presented to patients (HHS, 2008). Nurses should be prepared to address HL concerns, especially as they relate to how patient health education is disseminated (Eadie, 2014). Integrating inclusive patient technologies into nursing workflows could result in the assured delivery of targeted patient education information and improve patient outcomes related to patient understanding and comprehension (Danis et al., 2014). Knowing health literacy statuses on all patients would allow nurses the opportunity to tailor educational interventions based on each patient's best learning methods (Danis et al., 2014). Studies have established that patients with lower HL levels are at risk for poor health outcomes and that technology can be an effective means to engage patients and improve health outcomes, especially about the understanding of health-related education being presented (Prey et al., 2013). Consequently, it is important to ascertain patient HL levels, especially as it pertains to patient use of health education related interactive and inclusive technologies.

The purpose of this quantitative correlational project was to determine to what degree a relationship existed between health literacy scores, measured with the REALM-SF tool, and patient use of the iPET system to view health education modules for telemetry patients at a 225-bed community hospital in the Southwestern United States. The clinical PICOT question for this project asked do adult inpatients (P) that use technologically assisted interactive patient engagement technology (iPET) for health education (I) versus a similar group that does not use the iPET for health education (C) show a higher literacy score on the REALM-SF tool (O) when assessed during their hospital stay (T)? The REALM-SF tool was administered to assess HL scores on all patient participants partaking in this DPI project. All patient participants were shown how to use the iPET system and the teach-back method was employed to assess patient understanding of the provided iPET instructions. Demographic data, including gender and estimated age, were also collected. The independent variable was represented as patient HL scores and the dependent variable was determined by the dichotomous outcome of whether the patient used the iPET to view health education modules, yes or no. This chapter reviews the problem statement and clinical question as they incorporate into the following components of the project: project methodology; project design; population and sample selection; instrumentation; validity; reliability; data collection procedures; data analysis procedures; ethical considerations; and project limitations.

STATEMENT OF THE PROBLEM

It was not known if health literacy scores, measured with the REALM-SF tool, correlated to adult telemetry inpatient use of the iPET to view health education modules when compared to a similar group that did not use the iPET, after both groups of patients were provided the same instructions on functionality and use of the iPET system. Only 12% of Americans are considered to be proficient in comprehending and applying basic health information presented to them as it applies to their health and healthcare choices (Kutner et al., 2006). Smith et al. (2018) found that mortality rates were more than doubled in persons with low literacy when compared to persons with higher literacy rates. The Institute of Medicine (IOM) recommends integrating health literacy assessment screening into healthcare HIT systems to measure the effects HL has on patient outcomes as well as to monitor the best interventions which will address HL deficiencies (IOM, 2004).

Technological advancements in healthcare have a direct impact on nursing interventions, especially those involving patient education techniques for the hospitalized patient (Huston, 2013). Patients with lower HL scores have poorer health outcomes and may be less apt to be engaged in technological educational interventions, measuring health literacy, a vital component to help identify which educational intervention techniques are most applicable for the patients' literacy level (Mackert et al., 2016). Before the completion of this DPI project, it was not known if health literacy scores, measured with the REALM-SF tool, correlated to adult telemetry inpatient use of the iPET to view health education modules when compared to a similar group that did not use the iPET, after both groups of patients were provided the same instructions on functionality and use of the iPET system.

CLINICAL QUESTION

The clinical question that guided this DPI project was as follows: Do adult inpatients (P) that use technologically assisted interactive patient engagement technology (iPET) for health education, (I) versus a similar group that does not use the iPET for health education (C), show a higher literacy score on the REALM-SF tool (O) when assessed during their hospital stay (T)? This project used a quantitative correlational design approach to collect the necessary data to answer the clinical question. Evaluation of the independent variable, health literacy scores, was measured with the REALM-SF tool. The dependent variable was determined by the dichotomous outcome of whether the patient used the iPET to view health education modules, yes or no, as verbalized by the patient.

The REALM-SF tool was used to collect data independent variable data of HL scores and the REALM-SF scoresheet was used to collect the dependent variable data, whether the iPET system was used for education, yes or no. All participating patients were administered the REALM-SF tool, and all were educated on how to use the iPET systems functionality. The PI utilized the teach-back method to assure all patients correctly understood how to use the iPET fully. For all patients that correctly demonstrated iPET understanding through teach-back demonstration, the patient was left to utilize the iPET, and the PI returned after about an hour to ask the patient if they used the iPET, yes or no, to view patient education modules. For all patients that could not initially demonstrate how to use the iPET via teach-back, the PI conducted a second review on patient use of the iPET with the patient, and then returned after an hour to question the patient as to whether the iPET was used to view health education modules, yes or no.

The purpose of this quantitative correlational project was to determine to what degree a relationship existed between health literacy scores, measured with the REALM-SF tool, and patient use of the iPET system to view health education modules for telemetry patients at a 225-bed community hospital in the Southwestern United States. A correlational design was used to determine if health literacy levels increase a patient's propensity to use interactive engagement technology, in the inpatient setting, to partake in viewing health-related interventional education videos. Correlational studies provide an opportunity to determine the strength and direction of a particular relationship between variables (Asamoah, 2014). Determining first whether a relationship exists leads to later investigate the causation of that relationship, through additional projects and studies (Asamoah, 2014). Since there were gaps in the literature regarding health literacy and patient use of the iPET for education, using a quantitative correlational design provided the opportunity to collect quantitative data and use that data to determine whether a relationship existed between patient HL scores and patient use of the iPET to view health education modules. The methodology and design were chosen with future considerations as to whether nursing could effectively predict the best methods to provide health education to patients with varying HL levels.

PROJECT METHODOLOGY

A quantitative methodology was chosen for this DPI project. A quantitative methodology was selected over a qualitative or mixed methods approach. Quantitative methodologic approaches are characteristically objective compared to qualitative methodologies, which are often considered to be more subjective (Austin & Sutton, 2014). When choosing the methodology for this project, the PI carefully considered which methods would produce more valid and reliable results with ease of replicability.

Qualitative methodological approaches limit easy replication of a project, as data analysis is difficult without expert working knowledge of the subject matter, especially in terms of assuring that the data is interpreted in the same manner (McLeod, 2017). Qualitative projects have a higher risk for diminished confidence of reliability and validity (McLeod, 2017). Qualitative methodology projects collect data through observation, interviews, or via the use of a tool that measures attitudes or opinions, such as a Likert scale (McLeod, 2017). Quantitative data is interpreted through the use of numerical statistical analysis, providing a more scientific, objective, and mathematically rational approach, to ultimately yield more precise findings compared to qualitative methodologies (Denscombe, 2010). Quantitative methodology projects collect data in numerical formats, which can later be placed into categories, ranked, or measured as a type of unit (McLeod, 2017). Numerical data, in a quantitative project, can be collected via a measurement tool (McLeod, 2017). This project collected data using both a collection tool and through direct patient questioning. The independent variable was obtained as patient HL scores were measured with the REALM-SF tool, and the dependent variable was collected by the dichotomous response of whether the patient used the iPET to view health education modules, yes or no.

Data collected for this project contained both nominal and dichotomous categorical variable data. Patient HL scores were collected in a numerical format, using the REALM-SF tool, with possible scores ranging from a zero to a seven. Responses as to whether the patient used the iPET for education were obtained as a dichotomous variable of yes or no and later converted to a binary variable format, with yes equating to the number one and a no response equating to a number zero. The format in which health literacy scores and iPET data was analyzed, aligned with quantitative methodology.

The purpose of this quantitative correlational project was to determine to what degree a relationship existed between health literacy scores, measured with the REALM-SF tool, and patient use of the iPET system to view health education modules for telemetry patients at a 225-bed community hospital in the Southwestern United States. Analysis of the numerical nature of the variables was conducted within the confines of the clinical question and purpose for conducting this DPI project. Patient HL scores, collected on all patients, were compared to whether or not the patient did utilize the iPET for educational intervention. The project outcome sought to determine if there was a correlation between the variables.

PROJECT DESIGN

This project comprised a correlational design, as aligned with the project's quantitative methodology. A correlational design within a quantitative project measures and assesses the statistical correlation, or relationship, between two variables

(Price, Jhangiani, & Chiang, 2015). This design was chosen over the other available design options since it best addresses the clinical question using results obtained through statistical analysis of quantitative data. The PICOT question for this project asked if adult inpatients, that used technologically assisted interactive patient engagement technology (iPET) for health education, versus a similar group that did not use the iPET for health education, show a higher literacy score on the REALM-SF tool when assessed during their hospital stay? A correlational design measures two variables to assess for a statistical relationship, with no effort to control the extraneous variables in the process (Price et al., 2015).

Since it was not known if health literacy scores, measured with the REALM-SF tool, correlated to adult telemetry inpatient use of the iPET to view health education modules when compared to a similar group that did not use the iPET, after both groups of patients were provided the same instructions on functionality and use of the iPET system, a correlational design approach was best suited for this project to determine to what degree a relationship existed between patient health literacy scores and patient use of the iPET for educational intervention. When investigating the best design approach for this project, a quasi-experimental design approach was initially considered. A quasi-experimental design is often used to evaluate the effectiveness of an implemented treatment, such as when providing an educational intervention to participants and most typically utilizes a pretest-posttest as part of the design (Price et al., 2015). This design type was not selected, since it would not apply nor effectively answer the clinical question.

Educational interventions are commonly measured using a pretest-posttest design, in which the dependent variable is measured before intervention and again after the intervention is implemented (Price et al., 2015). Although commonly used in some clinical nursing studies, there is a level of uncertainty with the pretest-posttest design type, especially as it pertains to internal and external validity (Knapp, 2016). One of the considered threats relates specifically to the fact that using a simple tool to test pre and post scores may reveal a familiarity to the participant, therefore making the test easier and improving the patient's score. The pretest-posttest design was not utilized in this project due to the somewhat simplistic nature of the REALM-SF tool and the likelihood in which patients would recognize the seven single-worded medical terms.

The REALM-SF tool is a survey comprised of seven single-word medical terms. For this project, the patient read each word aloud as the PI secretly kept track of the time. Starting from the top of the list, the patient was asked to read each word out loud going down the list. If the patient correctly pronounced a word in five seconds or less, the patient was given a point for that word. If the patient took longer than five seconds, verbally passed on the word, or incorrectly pronounced the word, the patient received a zero for that word. At the end of the seventh word, the points for each word were tallied, revealing the final HL score. A copy of the REALM-SF tool can be found in the Appendix (see Appendix C). The seven words on the REALM-SF tool include behavior, exercise, menopause, rectal, antibiotics, anemia, and jaundice.

All patients were administered the REALM-SF tool. The independent variable of the project was the patient HL scores and the dependent variable was patient use of the iPET for education, yes or no. After data was analyzed, two groups emerged; patients that did use the iPET for educational intervention and patients that did not use the iPET for educational intervention.

POPULATION AND SAMPLE SELECTION

The setting for selecting the population and sample was a single telemetry unit within a 225-bed capacity community hospital, located in the Southwestern United States. A project or study population is defined as a group of subjects in which an investigator is interested in studying (Rebar, Gersch, Macnee, & McCabe, 2010). For this project, the population was comprised of adult patients ranging from ages 18–89 years old. Patient diagnoses were not known to the PI at any time, but all patients on the telemetry unit were continually monitored with a cardiac heart monitor. The 29-bed telemetry unit was selected for the setting of this project, since there was adequate literature to support nurse education of cardiac patients, as was discovered during the literature review phase of this DPI project.

After obtaining Institutional Review Board (IRB) approval, project sample recruitment began and was conducted over one month, with onsite recruitment occurring approximately two days a week. Patient subjects were selected through convenience, or consecutive, sampling techniques. When using consecutive sampling, all participants that meet the inclusion criteria are selected until the desired sample size and the time limit are reached (Martinez-Mesa et al., 2016). A subset of the overall population was selected to comprise the sample, using inclusion and exclusion criteria guidelines to determine patient eligibility. Power analysis calculations for independent one sample t-tests, conducted prior to requesting IRB approvals, using a power of 0.7, an effect size of 0.5, with a significance of 0.05, revealed an approximate sample size of 20.25 patients (ANZMTG, 2018). In order to assure that an adequate number of participants were included in the IRB request; a two-sample independent t-test power analysis calculation was conducted using a power of 0.8, an effect size of 0.5, and a significance of 0.05, which revealed a sample size of 50.15 participants (ANZMTG, 2018).

Patient inclusion in the sample was based upon their voluntary willingness and consent to participate. Patient inclusion criteria included provisions based on the patient's age and the patient's ability to read and write in English. The REALM-SF tool does not have an approved translatable counterpart in any other languages, which provided this language inclusion factor. The sample for this DPI project included 21 adults within the age range of 18–89 years old who had been admitted or placed on the telemetry unit as either an observation or inpatient status. Patients that could not speak or read English were excluded from sample selection. Patients over the age of 89 were also excluded from the sample selection, as patients over the age of 89 are considered as rare, patients aged 90 and older are considered to be identifiable. They were excluded to preserve patient confidentiality and to minimize risk. Nonverbal patients or patients unwilling to participate or provide voluntary consent were excluded from the sample selection. Patients that were on any isolation precautions were not included for the sample selection, to minimize patient risk. A total of 21 patients agreed to participate. All 21 willing subjects were administered the REALM-SF tool to measure health literacy levels.

INSTRUMENTATION

The instrument used to collect data on patient HL scores was the REALM-SF tool. A copy of the REALM-SF tool can be found in the Appendix (see Appendix C). The REALM-SF instrument was developed with funding from the AHRQ. Permission to use this tool was granted to the PI and can be found in the Appendix (see Appendix D).

The REALM tool was first introduced in 1991 by Dr. Terry Davis, PhD and colleagues and initially contained 125 health words. The REALM was reconstructed in 1993 and was shortened to 66 health words (Alqudah et al., 2014). The REALM is the most commonly used HL test in healthcare, as the words contained are only health-related words (Alqudah et al., 2014). The REALM tool has been revised many times, yielding several different versions. The REALM-SF, one of the revised tools, is considered to be the most usable form found in studies (Alqudah et al., 2014).

The 7-word REALM-SF instrument was developed by Dr. Terry Davis, PhD and her team, as a revision to the REALM tool (Cornett, 2009). The REALM-SF tool was developed to provide investigators an opportunity to quickly and accurately facilitate studies in literacy assessment applicable to a variety of clinical scenarios, while reducing the time spent with the patient, thus decreasing potential risks to the patient (Arozullah et al., 2007). The REALM-SF tool has been used in health literacy studies for almost 20 years and offers a much shorter administration time at two minutes when compared to the REALM, which takes about six minutes to administer (Cornett, 2009). The REALM-SF is considered a test of patient recognition, to provide healthcare clinicians with an immediate and valid assessment of patient health literacy levels (AHRQ, 2016). The REALM-SF instrument is comprised of seven one-word healthcare-related terms and is considered to be both valid and reliable. Instrument validity and reliability will be discussed in the subsequent sections of the DPI project manuscript.

Administration of the REALM-SF tool began by providing patients with a list of the seven medical terms, asking the patient to read each word aloud, from the top of the list down to the bottom of the list. The seven medical words on the REALM-SF include behavior, exercise, menopause, rectal, antibiotics, anemia, and jaundice (AHRQ, 2016). For each word that the patient recognizes and pronounces correctly, the patient is given one point, for a possible maximum total score of seven and any words that are not pronounced correctly are given a zero score for that word, for a possible minimum total score of zero. If a patient takes longer than 5 seconds to say a word, the patients are instructed to pass on that word, and the patient will receive a zero score for that word. Patients are instructed that they can pass on any words in which they choose or are not familiar with and in those instances, the patient was given a score of zero for that word. Depending on the patient's score, patients fell into one of four categories or grade levels, representing an equivalent to a HL level (AHRQ, 2016).

Patient scoring of a zero on the REALM-SF equates to a HL level of third grade or below, indicating patients would most likely not be able to read lower literacy educational materials and would need repeated oral direction with educational materials consisting of illustrations or both audio and video demonstrations and discussions (AHRQ, 2016). Patient scores of one through three equate to a HL level to that of a fourth to the sixth grader, requiring low literacy level educational materials. Patients scoring a HL score of one through three may not be able to read prescription labels (AHRQ, 2016). Patients that score a four through six on the REALM-SF tool represent a literacy level that equates to a seventh or eighth-grade literacy level, in which these patients may struggle with most patient education material and would likely not be offended by lower literacy materials (AHRQ, 2016). The highest score, a score of seven, equates to a literacy level of a high school student. Patients scoring seven would likely be able to read and comprehend most of the patient education materials provided to them (AHRQ, 2016). It is essential for nursing to understand the dynamic between patient HL scores and patient use of the iPET for education, to understand the best methods to provide patient health education to patients with varying levels of health literacy.

VALIDITY

Validity reflects the accuracy in which a measuring instrument or tool provides information about a studied variable (Rebar et al., 2010). Validity is demonstrated if an instrument or tool accurately measures what it is intended to measure (McLeod, 2013). The validity of the REALM-SF tool focuses on measuring health literacy and how accurately it does so.

The REALM-SF tool has been validated by multiple studies as a reliable means to measure health literacy in patients (Alqudah et al., 2014). A study by Arozullah et al. (2007) found the REALM-SF tool to be a valid instrument that can be used to assess patient literacy in a variety of diverse clinical settings. The REALM-SF demonstrated concurrent criterion validity with the REALM parent tool, with excellent agreement between the REALM-SF and REALM instruments (Arozullah et al., 2007). The

REALM-SF instrument scores were found as highly correlated in both development samples with $r = 0.95$ and $p = <0.001$, and in validation samples, showing $r = 0.94$ and $p < 0.001$, which both substantiate the concurrent criterion validity (Arozullah et al., 2007). Additionally, the REALM-SF and WRAT-R have strong correlation with other literacy tools, such as the WRAT-R with test scores showing as highly correlated at $r = 0.83$, $p = < 0.001$ in field testing validation (Arozullah et al., 2007).

RELIABILITY

The reliability of a tool refers to how consistent the tool is when tested and retested multiple times (Heale & Twycross, 2015). Reliability is demonstrated when tools consistently provide the same results, demonstrating that the aspects being measured have not changed (Macnee & McCabe, 2008). Cronbach's a is most commonly used to determine if internal consistency and reliability exist within a measurement tool (Heale & Twycross, 2015). The simplistic nature surrounding the administration of the REALM-SF tool provides the opportunity to consistently yield accurate results.

The design of the REALM-SF instrument is the most usable in healthcare to measure HL, especially in terms of looking at the ease of administration (Alqudah et al., 2014). It is of the reasonable assumption that any nurse administering the REALM-SF would produce the same results as any other nurse administering the REALM-SF tool. The REALM-SF tool demonstrated strong test-retest reliability at $r = 0.97$, demonstrating strength in reliability as a tool (Alqudah et al., 2014).

DATA COLLECTION PROCEDURES

The data collection portion of this project, which includes the administration of the REALM-SF tool and implementation of patient instruction on the use of the iPET, was conducted over the course of one month at the selected 225-bed community hospital in the Southwestern United States. During that time frame, the PI would visit the same 29-bed telemetry unit approximately twice a week. The patient sample was chosen from the population based on inclusion and exclusion criteria as well as the patient's voluntary willingness and consent to participate. The sample for this DPI project included 21 adults within the age range of 18–89 years old who had been admitted or placed on the telemetry unit as either an observation or inpatient status.

Patient inclusion criteria included provisions based on the patient's age. Inclusion criteria for patient age included patients 18–89 years. Any patient under the age of 18 or aged 90 and older was excluded as potential sample participants. Patients over age 89 years were considered as potentially identifiable, even in the absence of collecting any other identifiable data. Therefore, patients over age 89 were not approached to participate in this project. Patients that could not speak or read English were excluded from sample selection. Nonverbal patients or patients unwilling to participate or provide voluntary consent were excluded from the sample selection. Patients that were on any isolation precautions were not included as eligible for participating, to minimize patient risks. Patients that had any sort of assistive breathing device that covered their mouth or impeded their ability to speak were not approached to participate in this project.

During each visit to the site, patient sample recruitment began when the PI met with the unit charge nurse at the nursing station. Steps were taken to maintain patient confidentiality at all times. To maintain patient confidentiality and minimalize risk, the project site IRB approved this project under the confines that the charge nurse would review the list of patients on the unit and apply the inclusion and exclusion criteria to that list, therefore only providing the PI with a list of patient room numbers for patients that fit the inclusion criteria. No access to patient records was necessary, and no access to the patient electronic health record was obtained. Patient names, diagnoses, and dates of birth were not known to the PI at any time. The PI did not collect any identifiable patient information. The number of patients in the eligible population varied during each site visit.

As eligible patients were approached to participate, a brief introduction as to the purpose of the project and participant expectations was provided. Patients were informed that they would be asked to read seven healthcare-related terms aloud. Patients were informed that they would be instructed how to use the bedside iPET, reviewing functionality and purpose of the device and system. Patients were informed that the PI would leave their presence after that instruction for approximately one hour and would then later return with one follow up question. There was not any disclosure of what the follow up question would be, as it pertained to use of the iPET for education, to prevent any patient interpretation for suggested use of the iPET.

All interactions took place in the patient private hospital room. Initial introductions and explanations of the study were reviewed with the patient. Patients were notified that this project was a doctoral student project with Grand Canyon University (GCU). Patients were informed that this project sought to determine the understanding of healthcare concepts as it related to an interest in patient healthcare technology, such as the bedside iPET system. Patients were provided the opportunity to ask questions before deciding to participate. Patients that declined participation were thanked for their time, and the PI left the patient room.

A project site IRB approved script was read aloud to all patients willing to participate in this DPI project before obtaining informed verbal consent from the patient. This step was completed instead of obtaining a signed written informed consent. The IRB approved script contained all of the elements found within the project site IRB's written informed consent to participate. This was a provision of the project site's IRB, allowing to obtain verbal consent in place of signed patient consent, to minimize risk and prevent the need to store and maintain confidential paperwork for seven years post-project completion. A copy of the IRB approved script is included in the Appendix (see Appendix F), altered only to remove project site identification.

When reading of the script concluded, patients were again allowed to ask questions. Verbal consent was obtained on all patients that agreed to participate, which was verbalized by the patient when stating out loud that they agree to willingly and voluntarily participate in the project. A total of 21 patients agreed to participate. All 21 willing subjects were administered the REALM-SF tool to measure health literacy levels after verbally agreeing to participate.

The REALM-SF consisted of two individual pieces of paper, one being the REALM-SF scoresheet (see Appendix B) and one being the list of words that the patient reads from (see Appendix C). REALM-SF scoresheets remained in possession of the PI while patients read aloud the list of the seven medical words. The PI would mark the appropriate corresponding score on the scoresheet as the patients read the list of words. Patients that did not correctly pronounce a word, indicated that they would like to pass on that word, or took longer than five seconds to correctly pronounce a word, were given a zero score for that word. Patients that correctly pronounced the word within five seconds were given a score of one point for that word. After the patient got to the bottom of the word list, the total score was tallied, revealing the patient health literacy level score.

Patient names were not collected. Patient scoresheets were identified with a randomly assigned patient number that ranged from 0001 through 9999. Scoresheet assignment was arbitrary, and no identifiable association could be made between the patient room number and the patient identification number after the PI left the patient unit for the day. Patient scoresheets contained the patient HL score and the collected non-identifiable demographic data, which included the patient birth year and gender. Additionally, the scoresheet contained a yes or no checkbox for which the PI appropriately marked as patients were asked whether they used the iPET for education. The date was collected at the top of the REALM-SF scoresheet. REALM-SF scoresheets, although lacking confidential or identifiable data, will remain in the PI's possession for a total of seven years, as required by the project site IRB. The scoresheets will remain locked in a safe with the PI having possession of the only key code.

After the assessment of health literacy scores was complete, patients were asked to provide their birth year and gender. Patients were then provided instructions for using their bedside remote to access the iPET system. The visual accompaniment that was used while educating the patient is included in the Appendix (see Appendix E). The project site name was removed from the version in the Appendix. Patients were encouraged to follow along on their remote during the implementation of the iPET instructions. The PI pointed out the various aspects of the handheld remote, reiterating the purpose and function of each button identified on the accompanying handout. Patients were encouraged to interrupt and ask questions at any time. Patients were instructed that the select button could be used to pause a video. Once the video was paused, the right and left directional buttons could be used to skip forward or rewind video. It was emphasized that the skip forward button does not function during educational video play.

Patients were shown the various options available from inside the main menu, which included the section pertinent to their patient hospital stay, the available options related to the project site, the entertainment and relaxation options and the PI ended with the options available regarding health education. The Learning &

Healing section housed the patient educational video library and the medication library. Patients were encouraged to look through the available health education videos pertinent to their health, illness, or disease.

The teach-back method was used to assess patient comprehension of the instructions provided by the PI. To assure that patients understood how to access the health education videos, patients were asked how they could look up information on the iPET system about their medications. Patients that responded appropriately were thanked for their time and left alone with the iPET for about an hour. The PI reviewed the process with any patients that could not provide a correct teach-back demonstration. When reviewing the process was necessary, the PI approached the key points by rephrasing the information. After the instruction steps were complete, patients were thanked for their time and left alone with the iPET for about an hour. After approximately one hour, the PI returned and asked the patient if they used the iPET, yes or no, for education. Patient responses were recorded on the corresponding REALM-SF scoresheet. When the data collection period ended, data was analyzed on the 21 participants.

DATA ANALYSIS PROCEDURES

This DPI project used a correlational design. This project sought to determine if adult inpatients that use technologically assisted interactive patient engagement technology (iPET) for health education, versus a similar group that did not use the iPET for health education, showed a higher literacy score on the REALM-SF tool when assessed during their hospital stay. Data collected was analyzed to determine if a clinical correlation existed between patient health literacy scores and patient use of the iPET to view health education.

Data collection surrounding the independent variable, of HL scores, was collected through personal face-to-face communication with patients as scores were collected during administration of the REALM-SF tool. Data collection of the dependent variable was collected through face-to-face inquiry, after patients had an opportunity to use the iPET to view health education modules. Dependent variable data collection was completed by asking the patient directly if they used the iPET to view health education. The dependent variable assessment, collected as a dichotomous outcome patient response of either yes or no, was obtained an hour after iPET instruction concluded.

The project's supposition that patients with higher literacy scores will have a higher propensity to use the iPET for education than those patients with lower health literacy scores was tested using comparative means analysis. The PI postulated that providing educational instruction on how to use the iPET would engage patients with higher health literacy scores to utilize the iPET for educational intervention because of an increased engagement and desire to improve self-care behaviors, when comparing patient use of the iPET for education in patients with lower health literacy scores. To assess the size and direction of the relationship between patient HL scores and patient use of the iPET for education a Pearson's correlation coefficient © was calculated using Statistical Package for the Social Sciences (SPSS) software version 25. The correlation between these two variables was positive and moderate, $r(19) = .417$, $p = .060$. This supports the postulation that HL scores are moderately correlated with patient use of the iPET. The results were statistically nonsignificant, but clinically significant.

Descriptive and inferential statistics were used to conduct data analysis. Descriptive statistics were used to analyze the mean health literacy performance of the entire group of patients, by gender and by patient use of the iPET for education. Literacy scores were correlated to use of the iPET for education using Pearson correlation analysis. Pearson Chi-square tests were run to test the relationships between categorical variables, such as gender and patient use of the iPET. Statistical analysis of descriptive frequencies was conducted for all the input variable information collected. Analysis of variable means was used to compare estimated age with patient use of the iPET and estimated age with health literacy scores. Statistical and clinical significance was determined for all statistical analyses.

Descriptive and inferential statistics were used to conduct data analysis. Descriptive statistics were used to analyze the mean HL performance of the entire group of patients, by gender and by patient use of the iPET for education. Literacy scores were correlated to use of the iPET for education using a Chi-square test. Chi-square test was used to determine if a relationship existed between patient health literacy scores and patient use of the iPET for education, thus helping answer the clinical questions, do adult inpatients (P) that use technologically assisted interactive patient engagement technology (iPET) for health education (I) versus a similar group that does not use the iPET for health education (C) show a higher literacy score on the REALM-SF tool (O) when assessed during their hospital stay (T)?

Inferential statistics, such as t-tests and correlational analysis, were used to determine key differences between HL scores with patient use of the iPET and with gender. T-tests and inferential statistics were used to determine if one group (iPET used versus iPET not used) statistically and significantly outperformed the other in health literacy scores. Statistical and clinical significance was determined for all statistical analyses.

Data analysis procedures began by inputting raw data into SPSS software as variables. Dichotomous output data, such as the yes and no responses provided when patients were asked if the iPET was used, were converted to a numerical format, where one equates to yes, and zero equates to no. The REALM-SF tool measures HL in a numerical format, therefore requiring no translation of format. Patient gender was coded in SPSS as a one for female and as a two for males. Patient estimated age was derived by subtracting the current year, 2019, from the patient stated birth year. The patient estimated age was added to SPSS in numerical format.

ETHICAL CONSIDERATIONS

This project was presented and granted for approval by the project site IRB and the IRB at GCU. This project was deemed IBR expedited by the project site IRB and as exempt by the IRB at GCU. The project site IRB approved this project in a manner that minimized patient risk. Steps were taken to maintain patient confidentiality at all times. This DPI project adhered to the key principles of the Belmont Report: respect, justice, and beneficence listed within the basic ethical principles for conducting human research (The National Commission for the Protection of Human Subjects of Biomedical and Behavioral Research [NCPHSBBR], 1979).

To adhere to HIPAA guidelines and maintain patient confidentiality, patient protected health information was not disclosed to the PI at any time. The charge nurse was beneficial in assuring patient confidentiality was maintained at all time, as the charge nurse would review a list of the patient population on the telemetry unit and apply the inclusion and exclusion criteria to that list, only providing the PI with a list of patient room numbers for patients that fit the inclusion criteria and were exempt from the exclusion criteria. No access to patient records was requested, and no access to the patient electronic health record was obtained. Sensitive and identifiable patient health information was not collected at any time. Patient names, diagnoses, medical record numbers, or dates of birth were not disclosed at any time. All patients provided voluntary verbal consent to participate.

Respect for persons, per the Belmont Report, is defined as the respect given to an individual for their autonomy and the act of acknowledging patients that cannot represent their own autonomous decisions (NCPHSBBR, 1979). Respect for persons was adhered to as the PI treated the patients as autonomous agents, providing informed consent prior to obtaining verbal consent from all participants. Patients that had diminished faculties or that could not understand the informed consent were excluded from participation, therefore protecting patients that were diminished in their capacity to demonstrate autonomy. Beneficence is demonstrated when patients are treated ethically through respect for their patient decisions (NCPHSBBR, 1979). Beneficence was demonstrated when the PI respectfully accepted the patients' decisions not to participate in the project. Justice, per the Belmont Report, pertains to the benefits of research as well as the burdens participation brings to patients (NCPHSBBR, 1979). By adhering to the strict inclusion and exclusion criteria, the position of potential advantages or disadvantages of participation in this project were eliminated, assuring justice was maintained.

This project intended to improve patient outcomes for inpatients placed on a telemetry unit by assessing health literacy scores and correlating health literacy levels with patient use of bedside technology for health education. Conducted within the confines of improving the methods and delivery that nurses deliver health education to patients with varying levels of health literacy, this project maintained careful adherence to the key ethical principles of the Belmont Report: justice, respect, and beneficence (NCPHSBBR, 1979) for all patients during the delivery of providing patients with informed consent and while obtaining the patient verbal statement regarding their consent and willingness to participate. The three elements of informed consent: information disclosure, comprehension, and patient voluntariness (Thornton & Hipskind, 2019) were applied throughout the consenting process.

Patient consent to participate was provided verbally after the PI reviewed informed consent criteria with the patient via a project site IRB approved script. The project site IRB application originally requested permission to use a signed informed consent to participate, requiring a patient signature. The project site IRB made provisions to the original request for written consent, indicating that patient risk would be minimalized if an IRB approved script was read aloud to patients, which covered every necessary consent detail that would be otherwise found within a written consent. Topics covered in the script included the purpose of the project, patient eligibility, expectations, voluntary consent, risks, benefits, confidentiality, conflicts of interest, and cost. Patients were provided with a written copy of the site IRB contact information and encouraged to contact the IRB with any questions or concerns that were not addressed. Patients that agreed to participate willingly were asked to verbally state that they provide willing consent to participate in the project.

All collected patient data was consistently safeguarded. Patient scoresheets were identified with a randomly assigned patient number instead of collecting any patient names or initials. Scoresheet assignment was arbitrary, and no identifiable association could be made between the patient room number and the patient identification number. Patient scoresheets contained non-identifiable demographic data, such as the patient birth year and gender. REALM-SF paper scoresheets, lacking confidential or identifiable patient data, were stored in a locked safe and will remain there for seven-year periods following the completion of this project, at which time the paper scoresheets will be destroyed through a locked and confidential shredder.

Results from this project will be published through the GCU library in the form of a DPI project fulfilling the requirements for a Doctor of Nursing Practice (DNP) degree at GCU. No conflict of interest exists, and all HIPAA regulations were strictly adhered to during the entire data collection process. If any potential ethical issues arise, the PI will reach out to the chair, committee, and both the project site and GCU IRB, for guidance and support.

LIMITATIONS

There were several limitations this project. One of the limitations included the small sample size of 21 participants. Recruiting a larger sample from the population would be ideal. A larger sample size would have likely provided different results with more significant statistical results. Time constraints prevented more data collection opportunities. Another limitation in this project surrounded patient willingness to participate. It was difficult to find patients that were interested in participating. There are often difficulties recruiting patients in projects or studies, especially since patients do not emphasize the importance or scientific relevancy that clinical related healthcare questions may post to healthcare professions or health investigators (Sacristán et al., 2016).

A limitation existed surrounding the inclusion and exclusion criteria guidelines. A large potential patient population of 29 patients on the telemetry unit did not necessarily equate to all of those patients fitting the criteria for participation; therefore, making them unable to join the sample. Isolation patients made up patients within the overall population. Each time the unit was visited for sample selection, there were patients that were on isolation precautions, patients that did not read or speak English, patients over the age of 89, and patients that were disoriented. Additional barriers, not associated with the inclusion or exclusion criteria, included patients that were off of the unit for procedures or testing, making them unavailable for potential recruitment. This limitation is unavoidable as inclusion and exclusion criteria existed to protect patients from harm and to minimalize patient risks.

A potential source for an additional limitation existed with the confounding variables of the project. Confounding variables may mask or inaccurately demonstrate an apparent association between the intervention and outcome when no real association may exist between them (Skelly, Dettori, & Brodt, 2012). A confounding variable within this study could be that younger patients, regardless of their HL scores, may have an aptitude for using technology when compared to elderly patients. This is both uncontrollable and unavoidable. Patient estimated age was collected to potentially account for this concern during data analysis. Skelly et al. (2012) recommended to routinely assess the role confounding factors have in a project and to adjust for them accordingly during the data analysis phase of the project. Demographic data on age and gender are presented in chapter 4.

For this project, patients who used the iPET for education may have done so only because it was reviewed with them immediately before their being left alone for an hour, regardless of what their HL score was. Although the purpose of the intervention of iPET use for education was used to determine if patient health literacy scores correlated to that use, there may be an area of potential bias in that the patient may have used the iPET for education based on a suggestion from recent demonstration and instruction of how and why the iPET is used. In the absence of any intervention by the PI, patients may not have utilized the iPET for education at all during their hospital stay, regardless of their HL level. It is a minimal limitation, but one worth consideration and mention. One cannot determine what a patient would or would not do at any given point entirely, and therefore if this did occur, it was unavoidable.

SUMMARY

Low health literacy levels equate to diminished patient outcomes. Nurses should consistently be prepared to address HL concerns, especially in regards to how health education is provided to patients (Eadie, 2014). Knowing HL statuses on all patients would allow nursing the opportunity to tailor educational interventions based on each patient's best learning methods (Danis et al., 2014). Integrating inclusive patient technologies into nursing workflows could result in the assured delivery of targeted patient education information and improve patient outcomes related to patient understanding and comprehension (Danis et al., 2014). The PI's DPI project involved measuring patient health literacy scores, the implementation of providing patients with education on how to use the iPET and measuring the outcome of patient use of the iPET to correlate if a relationship exists between patient health literacy and patient use of the interventional iPET system to view education modules.

In this chapter, the methodology utilized for this DPI project was presented and discussed. This project used a quantitative methodology with correlational design. Quantitative data, interpreted through the use of numerical statistical analysis, provides a more scientific, objective, and mathematically rational approach (Denscombe, 2010). Using quantitative methodology allows for a more accurate determination of whether a correlation or relationship exists between patient health literacy scores use of the iPET for education.

Gaps in the literature, regarding HL and patient use of the iPET for education, supported the use of a correlational design. A correlational design provided the foundation to determine whether there was a relationship between patient health literacy scores and patient use of the iPET to view health education modules. This is an important consideration for nursing, as nursing seeks to improve patient outcomes by effective determination of the best methods to provide health education to patients with varying health literacy levels.

The REALM-SF tool was used to measure HL scores in this project. This tool is proven as both valid and reliable (Arozullah et al., 2007). The REALM-SF was developed to conduct quickly and accurately assessments of HL (Arozullah et al., 2007). The REALM-SF has been used in a variety of clinical scenarios for nearly 20 years (Cornett, 2009).). The quick and efficient manner in which the tool can be used reduces time spent with the patient, thus decreasing potential risks to the patient (Arozullah et al., 2007). Permission to use the tool was granted by Dr. Terry Davis, PhD, and a copy of the tool can be found in the Appendix (see Appendix C).

Data collection techniques and data analysis procedures were described in detail, with the expectation that other investigators would be able to replicate this DPI project. The unit charge nurse applied inclusion and exclusion criteria to the list of patients on a 29-bed telemetry unit. Patient protected health information was never revealed or collected. Patients fitting within the confines of the inclusion and exclusion criteria were approached and asked to participate in the project. Patients willing to participate provided verbal informed consent.

All patient participants were administered the REALM-SF tool to measure health literacy. All patient participants were provided a demonstration as to the function and use for the iPET. The teach-back method was used to assure patient comprehension of instructions presented to them. Patients were approached again after about an hour and asked if they used the iPET to view education modules. Data was collected and analyzed.

Data analysis was conducted with SPSS 25 software. Descriptive and inferential statistics were used to conduct data analysis. Descriptive statistics were used to analyze the mean health literacy performance of the entire group. Literacy scores were correlated using a Chi-square test to determine if a relationship exists between patient health literacy scores and patient use of the iPET for education, thus helping answer the clinical questions, do adult inpatients, that use technologically assisted interactive patient engagement technology (iPET) for health education, versus a similar group that does not use the iPET for health education, show a higher literacy score on the REALM-SF tool when assessed during their hospital stay? t-tests and correlational analysis were used to determine key differences between HL scores and gender. t-tests and inferential statistics were used to determine if one group (iPET used versus iPET not used) statistically and significantly outperformed the other in health literacy scores. Statistical and clinical significance was determined for all statistical analyses.

Ethical considerations were discussed pertaining to this DPI project. Adherence to HIPAA guidelines was followed at all times. Patient confidentiality and privacy were maintained at all times. The principles of the Belmont Report were consistently observed during the course of this project. No identifiable patient information was viewed or collected. No identifiable data was collected, and all statistical data was safely stored in a password protected and encrypted laptop. All paper data, which contained no traceable or identifiable information, was secured in a locked safe and will remain there for a period of seven years.

Limitations, relevant to this DPI project, were presented. Limitations in sample sizes, patient willingness to participate and concerns with confounding factors were offered. An explanation of each limitation was provided. The next chapter, Chapter 4, summarizes the data collected through data analysis and the reporting of results. Chapter 4 presents insight into the descriptive data, data analysis procedures, and results of analysis used in this DPI project. The analysis of the data and the results of the data are presented and thoroughly explained.

CHAPTER 4: Data Analysis and Results

Chapter 4 presents the data analysis and results. This direct practice improvement (DPI) project was designed to answer a clinical PICOT question. The PICOT question asked in this project was: Do adult inpatients (P) that use technologically assisted interactive patient engagement technology (iPET) for health education (I) versus a similar group that does not use the iPET for health education (C) show a higher literacy score on the REALM-SF tool (O) when assessed during their hospital stay (T)? The problem statement for this project was: it was not known if health literacy scores, measured with the REALM-SF tool, correlated to adult telemetry inpatient use of the iPET to view health education modules when compared to a similar group that did not use the iPET, after both groups of patients were provided the same instructions on functionality and use of the iPET system.

This DPI project was conducted on a 29-bed telemetry unit at a 225-bed community hospital located in the Southwestern United States. A quantitative methodology with a correlational design was utilized. The independent variable was the HL scores, measured with the REALM-SF instrument and the dependent variable was the dichotomous outcome of whether the patient used the iPET for education, yes or no. Pearson Correlation analyses were used to determine if there was a correlation between the variables and to help answer whether health literacy scores affected the incidence of patient utilization of bedside technology, the iPET, to view education modules after instruction was provided on the functionality and purpose of the iPET. A t-test analysis was conducted to determine significant differences between the health literacy measurements of the two groups, such as the HL scores between patients that did and did not use the iPET. This chapter summarizes the data collected and explains how the data was statistically analyzed. The results of those analyses are presented and described herein in this chapter.

DESCRIPTIVE DATA

The population for this project was comprised of adult patients, ages 18–89, who were admitted as an inpatient or observation patient, to a single 29-bed telemetry unit within a 225-bed community hospital. A subset of the overall population was selected to comprise the sample size, based on inclusion and exclusion criteria and patient willingness granted by a verbal informed consent to participate. The sample for this project consisted of 21 patients who were admitted to the same telemetry unit.

The design for this project was a correlational design. All 21 patient participants were screened with the REALM-SF tool to measure health literacy (HL) scores. All 21 participants were instructed how to use the iPET system and provided proof of instruction comprehension through the teach-back method. Following approval from both the site and GCU IRB, visits to the same telemetry unit occurred twice a week for a month until the data collection time limit expired, leaving the total sample size as 21. After the data collection ceased, data were reviewed, and patients were divided into two groups: those that used the iPET for education and those that did not use the iPET for education. Patient HL scores and patient use of the iPET for education were correlated, to determine if a relationship existed between the two variables; health literacy and use of the iPET to view education modules. Additionally, HL scores were compared against demographic data, such as gender, to discover if there were any significant findings in HL scores between males and females.

Descriptive statistical data derived from the 21-patient sample, revealed that most patients had a health literacy score of seven (66.7%), were female (52.4%) and did use the iPET for education (52.4%). The patient sample was divided into two groups; those that did use the iPET to view education modules (n = 11) and those that did not (n = 10). The mean HL score was 6.24 (SD = 1.26) (n = 21). For a sample size of 21 patients, 66.7% (n = 14) scored a HL score of seven, 9.5% (n = 2) scored a six, 9.5% (n = 2) scored a five, 9.5% (n = 2) scored a four, and 4.8% (n = 1) scored a three. There were no instances of patients scoring anything less than a three on the REALM-SF.

The estimated age range for the overall sample (n= 21) was 24–88 years old. The mean estimated age was 57.57 (SD = 17.63) (n = 21). The highest percentages of patients in the sample were 70–79 years. Figure 1 represents the percentage of patient participants in the sample based on estimated age ranges.

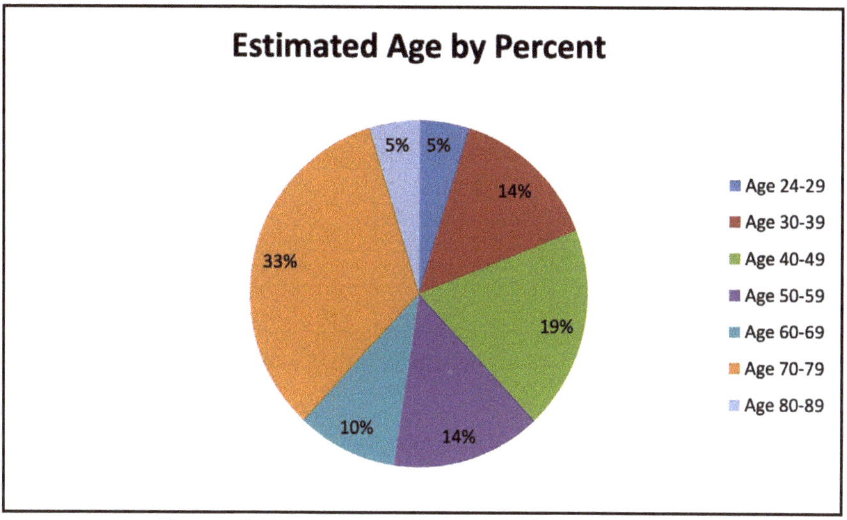

Figure 1. Represented Estimated Age Groups in the Sample by Percentage

Thirty-three percent of the sample (n = 7) was aged 70–79 years old. Patients aged 40–49 comprised 19% (n = 4) and made up the second largest age group. The smallest Age groups were both the 24–29-year-olds (n = 1) and the 80–89-year-olds (n = 1).

Of the 11 patients in the group that did use the iPET for education, 64% were female (n = 7) and 36% were male (n = 4). Analysis of data revealed that female patients were 1.75 times more likely to use the iPET than males. The estimated age range for patients that did use the iPET for education was 35–74 years old, and the average age was 54.54 years old (n = 11). The mean HL score for patients that did use the iPET was 6.73 (SD = .647) (n = 11). Of the 10 patients in the group that did not use the iPET for education, 40% (n = 4) were female, and 60% were male (n = 6). The age range for patients that did not use the iPET was 24–89 years old (n = 10), and the average age was 61 years old (n = 10). The mean HL score for patients that did not use the iPET was 5.70 (SD = 1.567) (n = 10). See Table 1 for a representation of the descriptive statistics for various demographic variables.

Demographic Variable Means

Measure	Males *M (SD)*	Females *M (SD)*	iPET used yes *M (SD)*	iPET used no *M (SD)*
HL scores	5.50 (1.51)	6.91 (.302)	6.73 (.647)	5.70 (1.56)
Estimated Age	56.10 (16.63)	58.91 (19.20)	54.45 (14.46)	61 (20.82)

Table 1. Demographic Variable Means

In order to discover if the demographic variables had an influence on health literacy, the patient sample was divided into two groups based on gender. Eleven females and 10 males comprised the sample size (n = 21). Table 1 highlights the means and standard deviation for HL scores and patient estimated age based on gender groups and patient use of the iPET.

DATA ANALYSIS PROCEDURES

Data collection commenced upon receipt of expedited Institutional Review Board (IRB) approval from the site and exempt IRB approval from GCU (see Appendix A). The data collection process occurred over an approximate one-month period. Upon completion of the data collection period, the data was retrieved and extrapolated from unidentifiable patient REALM-SF scoresheets. Data on the health literacy scores of all patients was analyzed. Patients were divided into two groups; patients that did use the iPET for education and patients who did not use the iPET for education. Additional analysis factoring looked at data relevant to patients divided into two groups by gender. SPSS version 25 software was utilized to conduct data analysis.

Data surrounding the independent variable, HL scores, was collected through personal face-to-face communication with patients during administration of the REALM-SF tool. Data surrounding the dependent variable was collected through personal face-to-face communication with the patient after patients had a chance to view educational videos through the iPET. Dependent variable data collection was completed by asking the patient directly if they used the iPET to view health education and recording patient responses. The dependent variable assessment, collected as a dichotomous outcome patient response of either yes or no, was obtained an hour after iPET instruction concluded. The independent variable was the patient health literacy score, measured with the REALM-SF tool, and the dependent data was whether the patient used the iPET.

Raw data was input into SPSS software. The variables collected included nominal and ordinal data, consisting of numerical data such as patient HL scores and patient estimated age as well as categorical data such as gender and iPET use. Patient estimated age was determined by taking the patient stated birth year and subtracting it from the current year, 2019. Dichotomous data such as whether the iPET was used for education, yes or no, was recoded numerically, with a zero input for a no response and an input of the numeral one for a yes response. Categorical variables, such as patient gender, were recoded from male and female into the numerical format, with the female being replaced with the number one and male being replaced with the number two.

The clinical question that guided this DPI project asked: Do adult inpatients (P) that use technologically assisted interactive patient engagement technology (iPET) for health education (I) versus a similar group that does not use the iPET for health education (C) show a higher literacy score on the REALM-SF tool (O) when assessed during their hospital stay (T)? Analysis of variable means was conducted to help answer the clinical question, as the mean for health literacy of each of the two groups: iPET users and non iPET users, was compared to determine which group statistically outperformed the other on the REALM-SF tool. An independent t-test was conducted to determine if there was any statistical significance to the difference in findings between health literacy score and the two patient groups as it pertained to patient use of the iPET. Correlational statistics were conducted to help answer the clinical question. Pearson correlations were used to determine what type of linear relationship existed between HL scores and patient use of the iPET for education as well as what type of linear relationship, if any, existed between patient HL scores when compared to patient gender groups. Statistical analysis of descriptive frequencies was conducted for all the input variable information collected.

Careful consideration was given to identify potential sources of error during the analysis of the data. Errors of statistical analysis, which can lead to incorrect assumptions and conclusions, are a potential risk during the data analysis phase (Brown, Kaiser, & Allison, 2018). A common type of error occurs in statistical analysis occurs when the wrong values are used in calculations (Brown et al., 2018). To assure the reliability and validity of the data calculations, human error was considered as a potential risk to data analysis. All data entered into SPSS was checked and double-checked to assure that the data entered matched the data on each of the REALM-SF spreadsheets. This was conducted to assure that the data was transferred correctly and without error. Results derived from data analysis are presented.

RESULTS

Health literacy scores were collected on all patients in the sample (n = 21). All patients in the sample were educated on the instructions for patient use of the iPET and all patients successfully used the teach-back method to demonstrate the effectiveness of iPET instruction. All patients were revisited after about one hour and asked if they used the iPET system to view educational videos. Patients responded with either a yes or no answer and that data was collected, coded, and analyzed.

For this quantitative correlational project, a single PICOT question was posed. The question was: Do adult inpatients (P) that use technologically assisted interactive patient engagement technology (iPET) for health education (I) versus a similar group that does not use the iPET for health education (C) show a higher literacy score on the REALM-SF tool (O) when assessed during their hospital stay (T)? Data obtained from administering the REALM-SF tool and through a face-to-face discussion with patients helped answer the clinical question. Data pertinent to answering the clinical question was analyzed in SPSS version 25 by comparing the mean HL scores of patients in two groups, those that used the iPET for education and those that did not use the iPET for education. T-tests were conducted to determine statistical relevance to any differences discovered in the HL means between the two groups; patients that did use the iPET for education and patients that did not use the iPET for education. Additionally, Pearson correlation was used to determine whether there was a correlation, or relationship, between the variables of health literacy and patient use of the iPET for education.

Using comparative means, data results showed the mean health literacy score for patients who did not use the iPET for education (n = 10) as 5.70 (SD = 1.567) and the mean HL score for patients that did use the iPET for education (n = 11) as 6.73

(SD = 0.647). These results demonstrate that patients, who did use the iPET for health education, did score higher in HL, as measured by the REALM-SF instrument when compared to patients who did not use the iPET for education. Zero is the lowest possible score a patient could potentially receive on the REALM-SF tool, and the highest score possible a patient could receive was a seven. The difference in HL score means is 1.03, which is a notable difference on an 8-point scale that measures from 0–7, so an independent paired samples t-test was conducted to determine the significance of that difference. Table 2 presents the independent t-test results comparing Health Literacy (HL) mean scores by group of patients that did or did not use the iPET.

t-Test for Health Literacy Scores by iPET Groups

	Independent *t*-test		
	t	*df*	*p*
HL	-2.004	19.00	0.60

Table 2. T-test for Health Literacy Scores by iPET Groups

There was not a statistically significant difference in the scores for HL and patients who did use of the iPET for education (M = 6.730, SD = .647, N = 11) and patients who did not use the iPET for education (M = 5.700, SD = 1.567, N = 10); t(19) = -2.004, p = 0.60, two-tailed. This result denotes statistically nonsignificant results when significance is deemed at $p < 0.05$. However, the p-value results do not determine clinical significance. Results indicate that there was a statistically nonsignificant, but clinically significant, difference in health literacy scores between the two groups of patients. Overall higher health literacy scores were noted in the group that did use the iPET for education by a score greater than one point.

Additionally, to help answer the clinical question, data analysis was conducted to determine if there was any linear relationship between patient health literacy scores and patient use of the iPET for education. To assess the size and direction of the relationship between patient health literacy scores and patient use of the iPET for education, a Pearson's correlation coefficient (r) was calculated (Table 3).

Pearson Correlation Matrix of HL Scores and iPET Use

	Literacy Score	*M*	*SD*
iPET	.417	6.24	1.26
	.60		
	5.38		
	.269		

Table 3. Pearson Correlation Matrix of HL Scores and iPET Use

The correlation between these two variables was positive and moderate, r(19) = .417, p = .060. This supports the supposition that HL scores are moderately correlated with patient use of the iPET. The results were statistically nonsignificant but were found to be clinically significant.

Demographic variables, such as gender, were used to conduct additional analyses, in an effort to discover if any relevant findings could be extrapolated from the data. The mean HL score for males (n = 10) was 5.50 (SD = 1.509) and the mean health literacy score for females (n = 11) was 6.91 (SD = .302). The difference in mean HL scores between males and female was 1.41, showing that women scored higher than men on HL scores. Since that was a notable difference between the two gender groups, additional statistical analysis was conducted to define the extent of a relationship between the variables and to determine if those results were considered statistically significant. To assess the size and direction of the relationship between patient HL scores and gender, a Pearson's correlation coefficient (r) was calculated (Table 4).

Pearson Correlations Between HL Scores and Gender (N=21)

	Literacy Score	*M*	*SD*
Gender	.57**	6.24	1.26
	.01		
	7.38		
	.37		

**$p < 0.01$ (2-tailed)

Table 4. Pearson Correlations Between HL Scores and Gender (N=21)

The correlation between these two variables was positive and strong, $r(19) = .572$, $p = .007$. This supports findings that HL scores are correlated with patient gender, with females producing higher HL scores than males. The results were found to be statistically significant and clinically significant.

Since women tended to use the iPET 1.75 times more than men, a Pearson Chi-square was conducted to test if there was any significance to this finding. The Chi-square test was performed to compare the proportion of females using iPET with males. The proportion between female use of the iPET over males was nonsignificant, $X^2 (1, N = 21) = 1.17$, $p = .28$. Additionally, there was not any clinical significance noted to this finding.

SUMMARY

This DPI project sought to answer a clinical PICOT question to determine if adult inpatients that used technology assisted interactive patient engagement technology (iPET) for health education, versus a similar group that did not use the iPET for health education, showed a higher literacy score on the REALM-SF tool when health literacy levels were assessed during their hospital stay. Both nominal and ordinal descriptive and inferential data was collected and analyzed to help answer the clinical question as it relates to the purpose for conducting the project, to determine to what degree a relationship existed between health literacy scores, measured with the REALM-SF tool, and patient use of the iPET system to view health education modules for telemetry patients at a 225-bed community hospital in the Southwestern United States.

This DPI project was conducted on a 29-bed telemetry unit at a 225-bed community hospital located in the Southwestern United States. A quantitative methodology with a correlational design was utilized. The independent variable was the HL scores, measured with the REALM-SF instrument and the dependent variable was the dichotomous outcome of whether the patient used the iPET for education, yes or no. The clinical question asked, did adult inpatients that used technologically assisted interactive patient engagement technology (iPET) for health education, versus a similar group that did not use the iPET for health education, show a higher literacy score on the REALM-SF tool when assessed during their hospital stay? Results demonstrated that there was a statistically nonsignificant, but clinically significant, difference in health literacy scores between the two groups of patients. Overall higher health literacy scores were noted in the group that did use the iPET for education by a score greater than one point. Using comparative means, data results showed the mean health literacy score for patients who did not use the iPET for education (n = 10) as 5.70 (SD = 1.567) and the mean HL score for patients that did use the iPET for education (n = 11) as 6.73 (SD = 0.647). These results demonstrate that patients, who did use the iPET for health education, did score higher in HL, as measured by the REALM-SF instrument when compared to patients who did not use the iPET for education.

The purpose of this quantitative correlational project was to determine to what degree a relationship existed between health literacy scores, measured with the REALM-SF tool, and patient use of the iPET system to view health education modules for telemetry patients at a 225-bed community hospital in the Southwestern United States. In order to assess the size and direction of the relationship between patient HL scores and patient use of the iPET for education a Pearson's correlation coefficient (r) was calculated using Statistical Package for the Social Sciences (SPSS) software version 25. The correlation between these two variables was positive and moderate, r(19) = .417, p = .060. This supports the postulation that HL scores are moderately correlated with patient use of the iPET. The results were statistically nonsignificant, but clinically significant.

Results demonstrated that patients that used the iPET for education scored higher on the REALM-SF tool than patients that did not use the iPET. Pearson Correlation analyses were used to determine if there was a correlation between the dependent and independent variables and to explore the type of relationship, if any, was present between health literacy scores and patient use of the iPET for education. It was discovered that a moderate positive linear relationship does exist between patient health literacy levels and patient use of the iPET to view health education modules. To further accentuate on the findings of that relationship, t-test analysis was conducted to identify the difference in means between the HL measurements of the two groups and whether that difference was statistically significant. Findings demonstrated that the relationship was not statistically significant, but it was notably clinically significant, as there was a one-point difference in HL scores of patients that did and did not use the iPET, which is considerable on a 7-point total possible REALM-SF score ranging on a 0–7 scale.

Both statistically and clinically significant findings were discovered when comparing health literacy scores with gender. Results demonstrated a strong positive relationship between gender and HL scores. Females scored higher in HL than males and females were 1.75 times more likely than males to use the iPET, yet Chi-square analysis did not defend this finding with statistical significance. There was little support to defend clinical significance of this finding.

The next chapter, Chapter 5, will summarize the project comprehensively and in its entirety. The importance of using the REALM-SF tool to measure health literacy will be defended and reiterated in Chapter 5. The contributions this project bring to the existing body of knowledge as well as the merits and recommendations for screening all patients with the REALM-SF to determine HL levels will be clarified and discussed in depth in Chapter 5. Additionally, future plans for dissemination of the findings discovered during this project will be discussed in Chapter 5.

CHAPTER 5:
Summary, Conclusions, and Recommendations

Inadequate health literacy is of ubiquitous concern. Only 12% of the population in the United States is considered proficient in HL, leaving 88% of the American population as unable to effectively understand or comprehend healthcare education or instructions provided to them (Kutner et al., 2006). This is particularly concerning since low health literacy levels are directly correlated with negative patient outcomes (Wickham & Carbone, 2013). Inadequate HL levels inhibit people from partaking in the most conducive health promoting self-behaviors and from making the best healthcare-related decisions (HHS, 2008). After adjusting for variables such as race, ethnicity, income, age, and educational background, HL in itself is an independent risk factor for all-cause mortality rates (Sudore et al., 2006).

Identifying patients with low health literacy levels can be useful as a means to predict negative health outcomes (Wickham and Carbone, 2013). The United States government has recognized the crucial considerations surrounding low HL levels, especially as they pertain to the use of health information technology as a means to improve patient communication in the healthcare realm as well as in the identification of disparities in health literacy (ODPHP, 2017c). Using HL scores as a predictive factor can help nurses identify a patient's capacity to understand the educational interventions being presented to them, especially as it relates to delivery via healthcare technologies (Rymer et al., 2018). Patients with lower HL scores may have poorer health outcomes and may be less apt to engage in technological interventions aimed at education (Mackert et al., 2016), such as an iPET systems. This is of concern to nurses that may rely on or assume patients will effectively utilize forms of technology that deliver health education to patients. Obtaining health literacy levels on each patient would be beneficial to assess the patient's capacity for understanding as well as help identify any areas in which the patient may need special considerations regarding the dissemination of health-related education (Loan et al., 2018). For this DPI project, the REALM-SF tool was utilized to measure patient HL scores because of the quick and effective manner in which it could be administered as well as for its proven validity and common applicability to all clinical healthcare settings and age groups.

SUMMARY OF THE PROJECT

This DPI project sought to answer an important clinical PICOT question. The PICOT question posed in this project asked: Do adult inpatients (P) that use technologically assisted interactive patient engagement technology (iPET) for health education (I) versus a similar group that does not use the iPET for health education (C) show a higher literacy score on the REALM-SF tool (O) when assessed during their hospital stay (T)? The project population, consisting of telemetry patients, was selected based upon the wealth of available literature pertaining to health education with cardiac patients. The sample was chosen based upon the inclusion and exclusion criteria set forth in the project. Expedited IRB approval was obtained from the project site and exempt IRB approval was obtained from GCU.

The independent variable, patient HL scores, were measured with the REALM-SF tool. Instructions were delivered to all patients regarding the use and functionality of the iPET. The dependent variable was whether the patient used the iPET for education, yes or no. Additional data collected included gender and estimated age. Data were analyzed using SPSS version 25. Pearson correlations were conducted to determine the extent and type of linear relationship that existed between health literacy scores and patient use of the iPET for education as well as patient health literacy scores with patient gender. Statistical analysis of descriptive frequencies was conducted for all the input variable information collected. Analyses with t-tests were conducted to determine significant differences between the measurement of two groups, such as HL scores between patients that did and did not use the iPET. Chi-square analysis was conducted to determine the statistical significance of findings as they related to females being more apt to use the iPET than males.

The purpose of this quantitative correlational project was to determine to what degree a relationship existed between health literacy scores, measured with the

REALM-SF tool, and patient use of the iPET system to view health education modules for telemetry patients at a 225-bed community hospital in the Southwestern United States. It should not be assumed that iPET technology would be the best interventional fit for all patients as a means to receive health education. The project outcome demonstrates that although the iPET was available, and patients were all provided education on how to use the technology, patients would not necessarily utilize that technology for health education; rather their HL scores would impact potential use of the iPET for education. Exploration of the clinical question was necessary to yield an outcome tailored to nurses that are providing health education to patients, especially through the use of technology. This chapter will present the summary and conclusions, implications, and recommendations stemming from this DPI project, especially as it relates to integrating the REALM-SF tool into nursing workflows and clinical practice, as a means to assess individual patient HL, to determine the best methodology for providing patient education based on HL levels.

SUMMARY OF FINDINGS AND CONCLUSION

There is plentiful evidence in the literature that outlines and identifies the correlations that HL levels have on patient outcomes. Low HL is considered a strong predictor for poor health outcomes, and is an identifiable risk factor for all-cause mortality rates, especially after adjusting for demographics such as age, race, gender, income, education, and health status (Sudore et al., 2006). The noted link between health inequalities and lower health literacy levels are identified within all demographic groups, yet there is a greater prevalence found in populations with chronic health conditions (Loan et al., 2018). Negative health outcomes stemming from low health literacy levels include decreased participation in routine health maintenance or preventative health behaviors, diminished success rates of patient self-care management in chronic diseases, and barriers to patient understanding of health-related education materials as they are presented (Wickham & Carbone, 2013). Low HL levels can prohibit the proper patient understanding and patient participation in educational interventions within an acute setting, as presented by nursing (Wickham & Carbone, 2013). Nurses often present as the primary assessor to gauge patient understanding of health-related materials and assess patient willingness to participate in their health maintenance, making nursing an integral aspect for identifying and preventing negative outcomes as they relate to a lack of adequate HL.

A single clinical question outlined this DPI project, as it related to the delivery of health education through technologic means while emphasizing the importance of identifying HL levels in all patients. The clinical question guiding this project asked: Do adult inpatients that used technologically assisted interactive patient engagement technology (iPET) for health education, versus a similar group that did not use the iPET for health education, show a higher literacy score on the REALM-SF tool when assessed during their hospital stay? Absent from the literature were studies specific to HL scores and patient use of the iPET for educational purposes. The specific findings stemming from this project, and conclusions based on analysis of the data will be conveyed subsequently.

Analysis of the data derived from this DPI project answered the clinical question. Health literacy scores and the incidence of patient use of the iPET for health education were accounted for during the data collection phase of this project. Data analysis, conducted using SPSS version 25, yielded results which support the clinical question, as data revealed that patients who used the iPET for health education, did score higher in HL, as measured by the REALM-SF tool when compared to patients that did not use the iPET for health education. Results demonstrated a statistically nonsignificant, but clinically significant, relationship between patient health literacy scores and patient use of the iPET for education.

Using comparative means, data results showed the mean health literacy score for patients who did not use the iPET for education ($n = 10$) as 5.70 ($SD = 1.567$) and the mean HL score for patients that did use the iPET for education ($n = 11$) as 6.73 ($SD = 0.647$). The difference in HL scores between the two groups is 1.03, which is a considerable difference in a HL measurement scale of zero through seven. Additionally, to help answer the clinical question, Pearson correlation was used to determine if there was a correlation, or relationship, between the variables of HL and patient use of the iPET for education. The correlation between these two variables was positive and moderate, $r(19) = .417$, $p = .060$. This supports the clinical question by demonstrating that HL scores are moderately and positively correlated with patient use of the iPET, therefore, as patient HL increases, patient use of the iPET would likely increase.

An independent t-test was conducted to determine if there was any statistical relevance to the difference in health literacy means between the two groups; patients that did use the iPET for education and patients that did not use the iPET for education. There was not a statistically significant difference in the scores for HL with patients who did use of the iPET for education (M = 6.730, SD = .647, N = 11) and patients who did not use the iPET for education (M = 5.700, SD = 1.567, N = 10); t(19) = -2.004, p = 0.60, two-tailed. Overall higher HL scores were noted in the group that did use the iPET for education by a score greater than one point. Results indicate that there was a statistically nonsignificant, but clinically significant, difference in HL scores between the two groups of patients.

The results are considered clinically significant because the findings are relevant to patient safety concerns related to the potential that patients with lower HL are at increased risk for misunderstanding health education materials. Assessing health literacy scores on all patients can help identify potential risks for misunderstanding as well as in the absence of knowing a patient's HL level, alleviate the assumption that all patients may benefit from the same methods of educational intervention. A score on the REALM-SF of four through six translates to the potential that a patient may struggle with most of the provided healthcare education written materials presented (AHRQ, 2016). Since the mean health literacy scores of patients not using the iPET falls in this range at 5.70, perhaps an educational video would be more beneficial for patients that cannot easily comprehend and utilize education disseminated in a written format, yet the group that could most highly benefit from obtaining education via the iPET, failed to utilize it.

Patients that did not use the iPET actually fall within a lower health literacy range than those that did use the iPET, thus placing these patients at increased risk for higher mortality rates (Peterson et al., 2011), higher readmission rates, and diminished adherence to medication (Rymer et al., 2018) than patients that did use the iPET. Nurses play an integral role in identifying, fostering, and enhancing HL (Loan et al., 2018). Because patients, who did not use the iPET, actually fall within a literacy range for which the iPET may best fit for them, stressed is the importance for nurses to measure HL scores on all patients, in an effort to properly tailor the dissemination of nursing education to patients aimed at the individual patient.

Demographic factors, such as gender, can influence self-care behaviors and impact patient engagement (Villarruel et al., 2001). Gender considerations are clinically significant, especially when pertaining to the engagement of patients in their own healthcare decisions through the use of technologies, such as the iPET. Not only is HL a predictor for patient outcomes, but active patient engagement is also associated with improved patient outcomes (Nunlist et al., 2016). Orem asserted that demographic factors such as age, gender, and sociocultural statuses could influence self-care behaviors and impact patient engagement (Villarruel et al., 2001). One of the goals of the iPET system is to increase patient engagement through the use of technology (Patmon et al., 2016). Nursing interventions aimed at education and guiding patient learning are vital considerations when addressing patient self-care deficits and patient engagement in their care (Orem, 1995).

Demographic factors, such as gender, were used to conduct additional data analyses, in an effort to discover if any relevant findings could be extrapolated from the data. The mean HL score for males (n = 10) was 5.50 (SD = 1.509) and the mean HL score for females (n = 11) was 6.91 (SD = .302). The difference in mean health literacy scores between males and female was 1.41, showing that women scored higher than men on HL scores. Pearson correlation tests were conducted and revealed a positive and strong correlation between gender and patient HL scores, r(19) = .572, p = .007. This supports findings that HL scores are correlated with patient gender, with females producing higher HL scores than males. The significance of these findings is supported statistically and clinically.

Clinically these findings are pertinent as gender can play a role in influencing self-care behaviors, which may ultimately influence patient use of the iPET. These findings explore the possibility that health literacy levels may be influenced by gender, therefore adding an additional consideration for nurses seeking to determine the best methods for disseminating patient education in an acute setting. Additional study is necessary as it pertains to health literacy and gender. This further emphasizes the importance of assessing HL scores on all patients. Further assessment and study are necessary to determine potential causation for why females tend to score higher in HL than males. If HL was measured on all patients and maintained as part of the patient record, data could easily be extrapolated from electronic health records for analysis to better understand the relationship between HL and gender; yet routine HL screening is not commonplace in the United States.

There is great emphasis placed on patient education and patient engagement with HIT, especially as it pertains to methods to improve patient outcomes (Cassano, 2019). The Institute of Medicine (IOM) recommends integrating health literacy assessment screening into healthcare HIT systems to measure the effects health literacy has on patient outcomes as well as to monitor the best interventions which will address health literacy deficiencies (IOM, 2004). The lack of a formalized process for nursing units or specialized care areas to routinely screen patients for HL levels is problematic, as nursing attempts to delivery patient health education to patients with different levels of HL (Loan et al., 2018). Additionally, nursing plays a crucial role in the integration of patient use of the iPET, especially for educational purposes, in the acute care setting (Patmon et al., 2016). As a means to improve patient outcomes, there is current and sufficient evidence to support measuring health literacy scores on all patients (IOM, 2004). Rymer et al. (2018) find that further studies are necessary to understand the effects that inpatient health literacy screening can have on improving patient outcomes.

Health literacy is recognized as a determinant of health outcomes (Logan et al., 2015). In order for nursing to foster positive patient outcomes, nursing must understand the barriers that may exist in patient attainment of improved or positive outcomes. To best understand the impact that HL scores have on patient understanding of the education that is presented to them, it is imperative to assess patient HL scores. Healthcare systems and nursing must work together to provide patients with the most optimal resources required for targeting patients with the best evidence-based methods to provide patients with education that is based upon what best fits patients as determined by patient health literacy scores (Loan et al., 2018). Studies demonstrate that hospitals routinely screening patients for health literacy demonstrated both lower readmission risks and higher compliance with patient prescribe medication regimens (Rymer et al., 2018). Since 2012, the Joint Commission has recommended that hospitals assess and document patient health literacy levels, yet this recommendation is few healthcare systems have adopted this advice (Rymer et al., 2018).

Using health literacy scores as a predictive factor can help nursing predetermine patient capacity for understanding the educational interventions being presented to them, especially as it relates to delivery via healthcare technologies. Patient use of technology within the acute setting is an important consideration when seeking to determine health literacy statuses. Patients with lower health literacy scores may have poorer health outcomes and may be less apt to be engaged in technological educational interventions (Mackert et al., 2016).

The purpose of this quantitative correlational project was to determine to what degree a relationship existed between health literacy scores, measured with the REALM-SF tool, and patient use of the iPET system to view health education modules for telemetry patients at a 225-bed community hospital in the Southwestern United States. This project identified the importance of administering the REALM-SF as an effective means to measure health literacy and that even though the implementation of training regarding the iPET occurred for every patient, not every patient used the iPET for education. The project outcome demonstrated that although the iPET was available, and patients were all provided education on how to use the technology, patients would not necessarily utilize that technology for health education; rather their HL scores would impact potential use of the iPET for education. An essential goal of this project was to strengthen the awareness of the impact that HL scores have on patient use of interactive technology for educational intervention, since iPET technology may not be the best interventional fit for all patients as a means to receive health education.

It is important for nurses to understand the dynamic between patient health literacy scores and patient education, so as to understand the best methods of disseminating health education to patients with varying levels of health literacy and to properly tailor the recommended education type to each patient, so that patients can attain the highest level of understanding in order to improve self-care behaviors and promote positive patient outcomes. Delivering targeted education to patients based on their health literacy levels is an important consideration, as patients may benefit from diverse types of educational materials, with emphasis of each based upon their health literacy levels as measured with the REALM-SF tool. The fact that not all patients may benefit from education presented through the iPET, stresses the importance for nurses to assess the health literacy levels of each individual patient.

This DPI project examined whether patient health literacy scores correlated to patient use of the iPET. Patients with higher health literacy scores were more likely to view physician prescribed health education videos through the healthcare technology iPET system, and results support that patients with higher literacy scores tended to use the iPET more than patients with lower HL scores. Not every patient will use the iPET or benefit from a form of technological education intervention, however nursing cannot even begin to explore the potential best methods of delivering targeted education to patients if nurses do not know the level of understanding that patient may have. Delivering healthcare education to patients based on their comprehension provides patients with the best opportunity to understand the education material being presented. This aligns with the ultimate goal to engage patients through intervention of patient education in order for patients to attain the highest level of understanding and comprehension that promotes positive outcomes and self-care behaviors for all patients. Instructional intervention was provided to all patients, since patient engagement and use of technology to improve patient outcomes is supported in the literature. Instruction was necessary as patients may not have been fully aware of the functionality of the iPET. Health literacy was a consideration in patient use of the iPET for education.

Exploration of the clinical question was necessary to yield an outcome tailored to nurses that are providing health education to patients, especially through the use of technology. Nurses cannot tailor education delivery to patients on an individual level without first having the knowledge of what that patient may be able to comprehend and in what form the education is best delivered. Ultimately, nurses seek to engage patients in their care and promote healing and positive outcomes for patients, often within short periods of available time to actually address patient educational needs. Capitalizing on the knowledge of health literacy levels allows nurses to save time in their workflow and maximize efforts so that patients can achieve the most optimal outcomes possible. Implications, especially as they relate to integrating the REALM-SF tool into nursing workflows and clinical practice as a means to assess individual patient health literacy, to determine the best methodology for providing patient education based on HL levels, will be explored. Practical, theoretical, and future implications stemming from the project will be discussed.

IMPLICATIONS

This project was conducted in accordance with the recommended practical and applicable uses for measuring HL with the REALM-SF tool. Noted results and findings from this DPI project have implications and applicability to the SCDTN, the theoretical foundation selected to support this project. Suggestions stemming from the findings of this project are presented with consideration as to any theoretical, practical, and future implications.

THEORETICAL IMPLICATIONS

The SCDTN focuses on the interaction between nurse and patient, so as that the nurse can determine a clear understanding of what the qualitative and quantitative values of variables are for both the patient and the nurse (Orem & Taylor, 2011). The clinical question for this DPI project asked: Do adult inpatients that use technologically assisted interactive patient engagement technology (iPET) for health education, versus a similar group that does not use the iPET for health education, show a higher literacy score on the REALM-SF tool when assessed during their hospital stay? Measured in quantitative values, the independent variable for this project was patient health literacy scores, and the dependent variable for this project was the patient use of the iPET for education, yes or no. For this project, interactions with patients occurred through communication that allowed for measurement of HL scores, the discovery of patient comprehension of instructions given on the iPET, and analyzation of pertinent findings to determine the impact that HL scores have on patient use of the iPET.

Under Orem's theory, nursing aims to assist all persons in need of achieving self-care, such as through the recognition and addressing of any internal and external factors that may pose as a barrier for patients which prevents them from addressing self-care deficits or needs (Villarruel et al., 2001). Findings from this DPI project identified a correlation between health literacy scores and patient use of the iPET as positive and moderate, $r(19) = .417$, $p = .060$. This supports and answers the clinical question through the finding that health literacy scores are moderately correlated with patient use of the iPET, suggesting that as patient HL scores increase, patient use of the iPET would likely increase.

Based upon the mean HL scores for patients who did not use the iPET for education ($n = 10$) of 5.70 ($SD = 1.567$), patients that did not use the iPET for education would likely find an increased benefit from its use since health literacy measurements between four and six on the REALM-SF tool equates to likely barriers with patient comprehension of written educational material (AHRQ, 2016). These barriers would make educational video material options ideal, but patients are left up to their own accord to view these materials. It is postulated that patients choosing not to engage in the use of the iPET were not engaged in technology, creating a barrier to achieving positive patient outcomes. It is not known if patient HL levels influence patient use of technology in general, patient use of technology for education, or overall patient levels of engagement, posing as an area of weakness to this project.

Within the SCDTN, nursing aims to recognize deficits and seeks to assist patients in overcoming those barriers so that patients can ultimately achieve improved or proper self-care behaviors. If one of the barriers preventing patient use of the iPET is lower HL levels, nursing cannot begin to address health literacy barriers without first assessing HL scores. One of the strengths of this project involves the findings that support the importance of measuring HL scores. It is imperative that nurses understand the dynamic between patient health literacy scores and patient use of the iPET for education, to understand the best methods to provide patient health education to patients with varying levels of HL.

Knowledge of patient HL levels would help nursing identify a potential self-care deficit related to a lack of comprehension to written education materials, allowing nurses the opportunity to engage patients through properly aimed interventions which target the best methodologies to approaching patient education and discussion. Nursing plays a crucial role in identifying and motivating patient use of the iPET (Patmon et al., 2016). Helping identify literacy deficits means nursing can approach patient engagement at a level tailored to health literacy and understanding, especially as it involves factors that can influence or improve a patient's self-care behaviors.

PRACTICAL IMPLICATIONS

When looking at patient perspectives regarding patient health literacy and use of interactive engagement technology, it is important to understand the effect that patient HL scores have on the use of the iPET for educational intervention. This project sought to identify and understand the best methods nurses can use to help provide health education to patients with varying levels of HL. The patient population selected for this project was done so in correlation with the existing literature pertaining to patient populations that have chronic health conditions. Assessing routine or standardized patient health literacy rates are not collected at the project site therefore, there was no existing HL data for the population being served at the study project site. A lack of existing health literacy data within this population allowed this project to learn of the relationship that HL scores have on patient use of the iPET for health education in patients with chronic health conditions. Patients admitted to a telemetry unit were assumed to have an increased potential for having chronic health conditions versus those from a patient population admitted to a general, non-specialized, nursing unit.

The purpose of this quantitative correlational project was to determine to what degree a relationship existed between health literacy scores, measured with the REALM-SF tool, and patient use of the iPET system to view health education modules for telemetry patients at a 225-bed community hospital in the Southwestern United States. The project outcome demonstrates that HL levels should be considered when predicting patient use of technology for education because all patients that were instructed on the use of the iPET and had it available for use did not all utilize it. The defining factor to consider was patient health literacy levels. Patients that scored higher HL levels on the REALM-SF tool did tend to use the iPET more than patients who scored lower on the health literacy scale. This finding stresses the importance that HL has on patient use of interactive technology for educational gain. A weakness of this project existed in determining the factors for which a patient may not use the iPET. Since patient diagnoses were not known during this project, it is difficult to assess whether factors such as chronic illness played any part in determining patient decisions to use the iPET or not use the iPET.

Assessing HL levels before educational interventions are offered may help nurses better understand the best avenues to provide educational materials to patients (Bullen & Young, 2016). The teach-back method was utilized and is considered a useful means to confirm whether the patient fully understood the material being presented, especially as it pertains to patient self-care behaviors (Bullen & Young, 2016). Practical implications stemming from this project stress the importance of knowing HL levels on all patients admitted or placed on the telemetry unit.

FUTURE IMPLICATIONS

The SCDTN focuses on the interaction between nurse and patient through communication and the exchange of information that pertains to both qualitative and quantitative variables, important to patient care (Orem & Taylor, 2011). Stemming from this project are recommended future projects, implicated in helping nurses gain an understanding of the factors surrounding patient self-care behaviors as they are integrated with HL, technology, and patient engagement. This is an imperative consideration for healthcare providers and nurses. Integrating HIT, HL, and patient engagement allows healthcare professionals to keep up with the best methods for engaging patients, educating patients, and directing self-care behaviors that will improve and promote positive outcomes (Huston, 2013). Health literacy levels can influence the degree in which a patient is engaged in their care, as patients that do not understand the pertinence of what is being explained to them will likely not be as willing to participate in the behaviors aimed at promoting or improving positive outcomes.

It is important to further explore and recognize why some patients are more engaged in their healthcare, why particular patients feel more comfortable with healthcare technology and identify how nurses and healthcare providers can educate patients in a manner that provides patients with the best level of comfort, so that they can better comprehend the implications involved with their healthcare choices. Potentially, this project creates a foundation for further projects involving the iPET and assessment of patient literacy scores. As a result of the findings of this project, further studies can seek to predict if patient openness to receive healthcare education through technology will identify early on those patients more prone to improving healthcare behaviors.

This project did help promote the national crisis and concern surrounding low HL levels while focusing on the methods in which HL relates to patient engagement in self-care behaviors and patient use of technology for health education. Future implications stemming from this project involve improving the understanding of how using technology may impact or improve HL scores as well as how findings and results may improve in significance through increased patient sample sizes. Assessing attitudes of both patients and nurses may prove beneficial to understanding the ways patient engagement, health literacy, and educational technology trifecta can improve patient outcomes and nurse workflows. Questions that may surround the REALM-SF measurement tool as being the best option for patients will need to be addressed to assure the best instrument or tool is being used, that minimizes patient risk and maximizes both nurse and patient benefits. Nurse practice considerations will be reviewed as it is applicable to recommended projects as well as to recommended courses of action surrounding the future practice.

RECOMMENDATIONS

This evidence-based DPI project accentuated the importance and impact of screening patients for HL levels. Patients that used the iPET demonstrated higher overall HL scores, yet the patients that did not use the iPET fell within a health literacy level for which the iPET would be most beneficial. It is the recommendation of the PI that all patients are screened for HL levels and that the project site implements the REALM-SF tool as a means to measure HL levels. As a result of the findings associated with this project, recommendations for future projects and practice, implications are presented.

RECOMMENDATIONS FOR FUTURE PROJECTS

This project used a quantitative methodology with correlational design. Using this methodological approach, health literacy scores were measured and correlated to patient use of the iPET for education. Results and findings from this project have generated additional ideas and concepts as recommendations for additional future projects.

One of the areas of the project that needs further examination is to look at the project from a differing perspective, such as to assess the role that the iPET may have on patient HL scores. Although the data from this project does support the relationship that patients with higher literacy scores have a higher propensity to use technology as a means to partake in healthcare education while hospitalized as an inpatient on a telemetry unit, there are gaps in this project. The project was not designed to identify if patient health literacy scores would improve after patients had the opportunity to use the iPET. Recommendations for a future project would involve completing a project of the same methodology and design type, but instead of measuring health literacy scores once, measure patient HL scores in a pre-test and post-test fashion, to compare if there was an improvement in the literacy scores after the patient had the opportunity to use the iPET and feel more comfortable with the technology format. Results of such a project could help support the permanent adoption of utilizing the REALM-SF to measure HL scores.

A limitation noted in this project involved the relatively small sample size of 21 patients. Time constraints prevented obtaining a larger sample size for this project. Repeating this project, but allowing for more time to acquire a larger sample, is a recommended future project concept. Statistical significance could be potentially proven if the sample size were to increase, as the larger a sample size is, the greater the possibility that the sample will accurately represent a population for which the interest is intended (Macnee & McCabe, 2008).

Utilizing a qualitative methodology project is another recommended project concept. The recommended project would involve measuring patient attitudes about interactive bedside technology geared towards health education and applying those findings to nurse practice workflows involving patient educational interventions. Additionally, qualitative projects surrounding nurse queries and health literacy assessment may be beneficial when considering recommendations that surround measuring HL levels on all acute care patients. Specific considerations involve working with nurses to inquire about their attitudes toward the assessment of health literacy scores on every patient as it pertains to integration into their clinical workflows and routine patient care. It is essential that nurses have confidence in the tools they are using to provide patient care and the opinions and attitudes of nurses are an imperative aspect to consider when implementing a workflow practice improvement initiative.

Since HL disparities are of national concern, additional projects involving health literacy and patient use of technologies for education would be recommended to assure those positive patient outcomes are achieved for patients with chronic conditions, such as those most likely to be found on a telemetry unit. A consideration and recommendation for a future project involve repeating the same project methodology and design, but instead of using the REALM-SF tool, use a different tool capable of quickly measuring HL, such as the NVS tool. The NVS survey was designed as a quick measure to formulate a numerical HL score based on the response to a series of six questions which relate to information printed on a nutrition label from a container of ice cream (Weiss et al., 2005). The

REALM tool focuses more on reading literacy as it relates to health, and the NVS focuses more on numeracy literacy (Shigaki et al., 2012). Assessing different aspects of HL can reveal additional findings or help support the validity of the findings in the pilot project.

Next steps in this project include recommendations for future practice ideas, based upon the practical and future implications deemed within this project. Practice considerations related to health literacy, workflow integration of HL measurement, and health-related educational technology, will be discussed. Project outcomes, as they relate to use of the iPET and effective communication will be explored.

RECOMMENDATIONS FOR PRACTICE

Disparities in access to health information, services, and technology typically yield decreased patient knowledge of chronic disease management and care (ODPHP, 2017a). Recommendations for future practice include applying a theory-based approach to nursing workflows that emphasizes and capitalizes on the important aspects surrounding Orem's SCTND. Integrating the principals of the SCTND into clinical practice provides nurses with the background and training to consistently maintain clear and concise communication with patients, especially as it is applicable to integrating HIT in patient care plans and nurse workflows. Nurses should constantly evaluate patient understanding, assess barriers in the achievement of patient self-care behaviors, and determine patient ability to comprehend what is being presented to them. Nurses that provide patient education or instruction should consider utilizing methods such as the teach-back method to determine if the instruction provided was adequate and conducted in a means that best fits the patient's comprehension or HL capability attainment of the situation. Improving patient HL and patient communication allows patients to understand learning material better and allow patients to make more informed decisions (ODPHP, 2017c).

The purpose of this quantitative correlational project was to determine to what degree a relationship existed between health literacy scores, measured with the REALM-SF tool, and patient use of the iPET system to view health education modules for telemetry patients at a 225-bed community hospital in the Southwestern

United States. In terms of this project, a key recommendation targets nurses that utilize or rely on iPET technology to provide patients with the means to receive their health education. Speculative assumptions based upon the findings in this project include clarification that nurses and healthcare providers should not assume that the iPET would be the best interventional fit for all patients as a means to receive health education. The project outcome demonstrates that although the iPET was available, and patients were all provided education on how to use the technology, patients did not necessarily utilize iPET technology for health education. This may be related to HL level, and although findings in this project support that, further projects and evaluations must occur. Although HIT is readily available to many Americans, it is not readily utilized because at least 50% of the adult populations fall within a low-level health literacy category (Mackert et al., 2016).

In order to understand the impacts that HL has on clinical practice in the acute care setting, it is imperative that health literacy is measured on patients during clinical practice in a hospital nursing unit. Exploration of the clinical question was necessary to yield an outcome tailored to the nurses providing health education to patients, especially through the use of technology. Integration of the REALM-SF tool, or an additional form of health literacy measurement tool, into nursing workflows and clinical practice is recommended, as a means to assess individual patient health literacy and determine the best methodologies for providing patient education based on HL levels especially applicable in scenarios involving patient use of the iPET for education.

REFERENCES

Adams, R. J. (2010). Improving health outcomes with better patient understanding and education. Risk Management and Healthcare Policy, 3, 61–72. doi: 10.2147/RMHP.S7500

Agency for Healthcare Research and Quality. (2016). Health literacy measurement tools (revised). Retrieved from https://www.ahrq.gov/professionals/quality-patient-safety/quality-resources/tools/literacy/index.html#short

Ahadzadeh, A. S., Sharif, S. P., Ong, F. S., & Khong, K. W. (2015). Integrating health belief model and technology acceptance model: An investigation of health-related internet use. Journal of Medical Internet Research, 17(2):e45. doi: 10.2196/jmir.3564

Ahlan, A. R., & Ahmad, B. I. (2015). An overview of patient acceptance of Health Information Technology in developing countries: A review and conceptual model. International Journal of Information Systems and Project Management, 3(1), 29–48. doi: 10.12821/ijispm03102

Alqudah, M., Johnson, M., Cowin, L., & George, A. (2014). Measuring health literacy in emergency departments. Journal of Nursing Education and Practice, 4(2), 1–10. doi:10.5430/jnep.v4n2p1

Alvarez, C., Greene, J., Hibbard, J., & Overton, V. (2016). The role of primary care providers in patient activation and engagement in self-management: A cross-sectional analysis. BMC Health Services Research, 16(85), 1–8. doi: 10.1186/s12913-016-1328-3

American Nurses Association. (2015). Code of ethics for nurses with interpretative statements. Silver Springs, MD: American Nurses Association.

Anderson, K., Burford, O., & Emmerton, L. (2016). Mobile health apps to facilitate self-care: A qualitative study of user experiences. Public Library of Science (PLOS ONE), 1–21. doi: 10.1371/journal.pone.0156164

ANZMTG.org. (2018). Power calculator for independent t-test or paired t-test. Retrieved from https://anzmtg.org/stats/PowerCalculator/PowerTtest

Arozullah, A., Yarnold, P., Bennett, C., Soltysik, R., Wolf, M., Ferreira, R., … Davis, T. (2007). Development and validation of a short-form, rapid estimate of adult literacy in medicine. Medical Care, 45(11), 1026–1033. doi: 10.1097/MLR.0b013e3180616c1b

Asamoah, M. K. (2014). Re-examination of the limitations associated with correlational research. Journal of Educational Research and Reviews, 2(4), 45–52.

Austin, Z., & Sutton, J. (2014). Qualitative research: Getting started. The Canadian Journal of Hospital Pharmacy, 67(7), 436–440.

Badaczewski, A., Bauman, L. J., Blank, A. E., Dreyer, B., Abrams, M., Stein, R. E., … Sharif, I. (2017). Relationship between teach-back and patient-centered communication in primary care pediatric encounters. Patient Education and Counseling, 100(7), 1345–1352. doi: 10.1016/j.pec.2017.02.022

Bailey, S. C., Fang, G., Annis, I. E., O'Connor, R., Paasche-Orlow, M. K., Wolf, M. S. (2015). Health literacy and 30-day hospital readmission after acute myocardial infarction. BMJ Open (5), 1–10. doi: 10.1136/bmjopen-2014-006975

Banfield, B. E. (1998). A philosophical inquiry of Orem's self-care deficit nursing theory (Doctoral dissertation, Wayne State University, Detroit, MI, 1997). Dissertation Abstracts International, 58, 5885B.

Baptiste, D. L., Mark, H., Groff-Paris, L., & Taylor, L. A. (2014). A nurse-guided patient-centered heart failure education program. Journal of Nursing Education and Practice, 4(3), 49–57.

Barr, P. J., Scholl, I., Bravo, P., Faber, M. J., Elwyn, G., & McAllister, M. (2015). Assessment of patient empowerment: A systematic review of measures. Public Library of Science (PLOS ONE), 1–24. doi: 10.1371/journal.pone.0126553

Baur, C. (2010). Calling the nation to act: Implementing the national action plan to improve health literacy. Nursing Outlook, 59(2), 63–69. doi: 10.1016/j.outlook.2010.12.003

Bennett, I. M., Chen, J., Soroui, J. S., & White, S. (2009). The contribution of health literacy to disparities in self-rated health status and preventive health behaviors in older adults. Annals of Family Medicine, 7(3), 204–211.

Berkowitz, B. (2016). The patient experience and patient satisfaction: Measurement of a complex dynamic. OJIN: The Online Journal of Issues in Nursing, 21(1), doi: 10.3912/OJIN.Vol21No01Man01

Bishop, A. C., Baker, R., Boyle, T. A., & MacKinnon, N. J. (2014). Using the health belief model to explain patient involvement in patient safety. Health Expectations, 18, 3019–3033.

Bluestein, C., Rothschild, D. B., Valen, A., Valaitis, E., Schweitzer, L., & Jones, R. (2014). Wait times, patient satisfaction scores, and the perception of care. The American Journal of Managed Care, 20(5), 3993–400.

Brown, A. W., Kaiser, K. A., & Allison, D. B. (2018). Issues with data and analyses: Errors, underlying themes, and potential solutions. PNAS: Proceedings of the National Academy of Sciences of the United States of America, 115 (11), 2563–2570. doi: 10.1073/pnas.1708279115

Bullen, B., & Young, M. (2016). When patient education fails: do we consider the impact of low health literacy? The Diabetic Foot Journal, 19(3), 138–141.

Cabellos-Garcia, A. C., Martinez-Sabater, A., Castro-Sanchez, E., Kangasniemi, M., Juarez-Vela, R., & Gea-Caballero, V. (2018). Relation between health literacy, self-care and adherence to treatment with oral anticoagulants in adults: A narrative systemic review.

Calvillo, J., Roman, I., & Roa, L. M. (2013). How technology is empowering patients? A literature review. Health Expectations, 18, 643–652.

Carman, K. L., Dardess, P., Maurer, M., Sofaer, S., Adams, K., Bechtel, C., & Sweeney, J. (2013). Patient and family engagement: A framework for understanding the elements and developing interventions and policies. Health Affairs, 32(2), 223–231.

Cassano, C. (2015). The right balance - Technology and Patient care. Online Journal of Nursing Informatics, 18(3), 1.

Cassano, C. (2019). Interactive technology is shaping patient education and experience. Journal of Nursing. Retrieved from https://rn-journal.com/journal-of-nursing/interactive-technology-patient-education-experience

Cawthon, C., Mion, L. C., Willens, D. E., Roumie, C. L., & Kripalani, S. (2014). Implementing routine health literacy assessment in hospital and primary care patients. The Joint Commission Journal on Quality and Patient Safety, 40(2), 68–76.

Centers for Disease Control and Prevention. (2016). What is health literacy? Retrieved from https://www.cdc.gov/healthliteracy/learn/index.html

Chahardah-Cherik, S., Gheibizadeh, M., Jahani, S., & Cheraghian, B. (2018). The relationship between health literacy and health promoting behaviors in patients with Type 2 diabetes. International Journal of Community Based Nursing and Midwifery, 6(1), 65–75.

Charlot, M., Winter, M. R., Cabral, H., Wolf, M. S., Curtis, L. M., Hanchate, A., & Paasche-Orlow, M. (2017). Patient activation mediates health literacy associated with hospital utilization among whites. HLRP: Health Literacy Research and Practice, 1(3), 128–135.

Charlton, C. R., Dearing, K. S., Berry, J. A., & Johnson, M. J. (2008). Nurse practitioners' communication styles and their impact on patient outcomes: An integrated literature review. Journal of the American Academy of Nurse Practitioners, 20(7), 382–388. doi: 10.1111/j.1745-7599.2008.00336.x

Chen, A. M. H., Yehle, K. S., Plake, K. S., Murawski, M. M., & Mason, H. L. (2012). Health literacy and self-care of patients with heart failure. Journal of Cardiovascular Nursing, 26(6), 446–451. doi: 10.1097/JCN.0b013e31820598d4

Christensen, D. (2016). The Impact of Health Literacy on Palliative Care Outcomes. Journal of Hospice & Palliative Nursing, 18(6), 544–549.

Cornett, S. (2009). Assessing and addressing health literacy. OJIN: The Online Journal of Issues in Nursing, 14(3), 1–13. doi: 10.3912/OJIN.Vol14No03Man02

Crowie, M. R., Anker, S. D., Cleland, J. G. F., Felker, G. M., Fillippatos, G., Jaarsma, T., López-Sendón, J. (2014). Improving care for patients with acute heart failure: before, during and after hospitalization. ESC Heart Failure, 1(2), 110–145.

Cutilli, C. C., & Bennett, I. M. (2009). Understanding the health literacy of America results of the national assessment of adult literacy. Orthopaedic Nursing, 28(1), 27–32. doi: 10.1097/01.NOR.0000345852.22122.d6

Cyril, S., Smith, B. J., & Renzaho, A. M. N. (2015). Systematic review of empowerment measures in health promotion. Health Promotion International, 31, 809–826.

Dalal, A. K., Dykes, P. C., Collins, S., Lehmann, L.S., Ohashi, K., Rozenblum, R., Stade, D., …Bates, D. W. (2016). A Web-based patient-centered toolkit to engage patients and caregivers in the acute care setting: A preliminary evaluation. Journal of Medical Informatics Association, 23(1), 80–87.

Danis, C., Ballen, S., Minniti, M. J., Farrell, R., Ball, M., Kennedy, R., … Yeo, S. (2014). Using technology to engage patients and improve outcomes. Journal of Healthcare Information Management, 28(1), Retrieved from www.himss.org/jhim/archive/volume-28-2014

Danvers, E., & Desai, R. (2008). Research ethics. Retrieved from https://study.cardiffmet.ac.uk/AcSkills/Documents/Research/Research_Ethics_elesson/page_10.htm

Deccache, A., & Aujoulat, I. (2001). A European perspective: common developments, differences and challenges in patient education. Patient Education and Counseling, 44(1), 7–14.

Dehbarez, N. T., Lynggaard, V., & Sogaard, R. (2015). Learning and coping strategies versus standard education in cardiac rehabilitation: A cost-utility analysis alongside a randomized controlled trial. BioMed Central Health Services Research, 15, 1–10.

Denscombe, M. (2010). The Good Research Guide: for small-scale social research (4th ed.). Berkshire, England: McGraw Hill. Retrieved from https://www.researchgate.net/file.PostFileLoader.html?id=582a0dbf217e20276533f5a5&assetKey=AS:428404664213506@1479151039119

Martinez-Mesa, J., Gonzalez-Chica, D. A., Duquia, R. P., Bonamigo, R., R., & Bastos, J. L. (2016). Sampling: how to select participants in my research study? Anais Brasileiros de Dermatologia, 91(3), 326–330. doi: 10.1590/abd1806-4841.20165254

Dunlay, S. M., Griffin, J. M., Redfield, M. M., & Roger, V. L. (2017). Patient activation in acute decompensated heart failure. Journal of Cardiovascular Nursing, 32(6), 560–567.

Eadie, C. (2014). Health literacy: A conceptual review. MEDSURG Nursing, 23, 1–13.

Ekenedo, G. O. (2015). Innovative applications of educational technology tools in nonformal and informal health education. In Adeoye, B. F. Innovative applications of educational technology tools in teaching and learning. Bloomington: Trafford Publishing.

Ellis-Jacobs, K. (2011). A Quantitative correlational study on the impact of patient satisfaction on a rural hospital. The Internet Journal of Allied Health Sciences and Practices, 9(4), 1–6.

Farahani, M. A., Mohammadi, E., Ahmadi, F., & Mohammadi, N. (2013). Factors influencing the patient education: A qualitative research. Iranian Journal of Nursing and Midwifery Research, 18(2), 133–139.

Fawcett, J. (2001). The nurse theorists: 21st-cenutury updates – Dorthea E. Orem. Nursing Science Quarterly, 14(1), 34–38.

Feudtner, C. (2001). What are the goals of patient education? Western Journal of Medicine, 174(3), 173–174.

Fredericks, S., & Yau, T. (2016). Clinical effectiveness of individual patient education in heart surgery patients: A systematic review and meta-analysis. International Journal of Nursing Studies, 65, 44–53.
Galanakis, M., Tsoli, S., & Darviri, C. (2016). The effects of patient empowerment scale in chronic diseases. Psychology, 7, 1369–1390.

Gallo, A. (2016). A refresher on statistical significance. Retrieved from https://hbr.org/2016/02/a-refresher-on-statistical-significance

Gammon, D., Berntsen, G. K., Koricho, A. T., Sygna, K., & Ruland, C. (2015). The chronic care model and technological research and innovation: A scoping review at the crossroads. The Journal of Medical Internet Research, 17(2), e25. doi: 10.2196/jmir.3547

Gee, P. M., & Patmon, F. L. (2016). Leveraging the power of ehealth. AADE in Practice, 4(3), 18–23. doi: 10.1177/2325160316639024

Ghisi, G. L. M., Abdallah, F., Grace, S. L., Thomas, S., & Oh, P. (2014). A systematic review of patient education in cardiac patients: Do they increase knowledge and promote health behavior change? Patient Education and Counseling, 95, 160–174.

Griffey, R. T., Shin, N., Jones, S., Aginam, N., Gross, M., Kinsella, Y., … Kaphingst, K. A. (2015). The impact of teach-back on comprehension of discharge instructions and satisfaction among emergency patients with limited health literacy: A randomized, controlled study. Journal of Health Communication, 8(1), 10–21. doi: 10.1179.1753807615Y.0000000001

Grondahl, V. A., Wilde-Larsson, B., Karlsson, I., & Hall-Lord, M. L. (2013). Patients' experiences of care quality and satisfaction during hospital stay: A qualitative study. European Journal for Person Centered Healthcare, 1(1), 185–192.

Heale, R., & Twycross, A. (2015). Validity and reliability in quantitative studies. Evidence Based Nursing, 18(3), 66–67.

Health IT.gov. (2013). Basics of Health IT. Retrieved from https://www.healthit.gov/patients-families/basics-health-it

Heath, S. (2017). How can healthcare professionals define patient engagement? Retrieved from https://patientengagementhit.com/news/how-can-healthcare-professionals-define-patient-engagement

Henwood, F., Wyatt, S., Hart, A., & Smith, J. (2003). Ignorance is bliss sometimes: Constraints on the emergence of the informed patient in the changing landscapes of health information. Sociology of Health & Illness, 25(6), 589–607.

Howard, D. H., Sentell, T., Gazmararian, J. A. (2006). Impact of health literacy on socioeconomic and racial differences in health in an elderly population. Journal of General Internal Medicine, 21(8), 857–861. doi: 10.1111/j.1525-1497.2006.00530.x

Hibbard, J. H., & Greene, J. (2013). What the evidence shows about patient activation: Better health outcomes and care experiences; fewer data on costs. Health Affairs, 32(2), 207–214. doi: 10.1377/hlthaff.2012.1061

Hibbard, J., & Gilburt, H. (2014). Supporting people to manage their health: An introduction to patient activation. Retrieved from https://www.kingsfund.org.uk/sites/default/files/field/field_publication_file/supporting-people-manage-health-patient-activation-may14.pdf

Hibbard, J. H., & Mahoney, E. (2010). Toward a theory of patient and consumer activation. Patient Education and Counseling 78(3), 377–381.

Hibbard, J. H., Stockard, J., Mahoney, E. R., & Tusler, M. (2004). Development of the patient activation measure (PAM): Conceptualizing and measuring patient activation in patients and consumers. HSR: Health Science Research, 39(4), 1005–1026.

Huang, Y. M., Shiyanbola, O. O., Smith, P. D., & Chan, H. Y. (2018). Quick screen of patient' numeracy and document literacy skills: the factor structure of the Newest Vital Sign. Patient Preference and Adherence, 12, 853–859. doi: 10.2147/PPA.S165994

Hull, S. (2015). Using technology to engage patients. American Nurse Today, 10(9), 13–14.

Huston, C. (2013). The impact of emerging technology on nursing care: Warp speed ahead. OJIN: The Online Journal of Issues in Nursing, 18(2), 1–14.

Ibrahim, S. Y., Reid, F., Shaw, A., Rowlands, G., Gomez, G. B., Chesnokov, M., Ussher, M. (2008). Validation of a health literacy screening tool (REALM) in a UK population with coronary heart disease. Journal of Public Health, 30(4), 449–455.

Ingram, R. R., & Kautz, D. D. (2018). Creating win-win outcomes for patients with low-health literacy: A nursing case study. MEDSURG Nursing, 27(2), 132–134.

Institute for Work & Health. (2016). Validity and reliability. Retrieved from https://www.iwh.on.ca/what-researchers-mean-by/validity-and-reliability

Institute of Medicine. (2004). Health Literacy: A prescription to end confusion. Washington DC: National Academies Press. Retrieved from https://www.researchgate.net/profile/Lynn_Nielsen-Bohlman/publication/303697782_Health_Literacy_A_Prescription_to_End_Confusion/links/574e41d208ae8bc5d15bfda9/Health-Literacy-A-Prescription-to-End-Confusion.pdf

Institute of Medicine Committee. (2011). The future of nursing: Leading change, advancing health. Washington DC: National Academies Press. Retrieved from https://www.ncbi.nlm.nih.gov/books/NBK209871/?report=reader

Ishikawa, H., Yano, E., Fujimori, S., Kinoshita, M., Yamanouchi, T., Yoshikawa, M., … Teramoto, T. (2009). Patient health literacy and patient-physician information exchange during a visit. Family Practice, 26(6), 517–523. doi: 10.1093/fampra/cmp060

Jacobs, J. (2015). How health IT can promote patient literacy. Retrieved from https://www.himss.org/how-health-it-can-promote-patient-literacy?ItemNumber=37910

Jarvis, C. (2013). Using technology to engage patients. Retrieved from http://www.healthcareitnews.com/blog/using-technology-engage-patients

JE de Veer, A., Fleuren, M. A. H., Bekkema, N., & Fracke, A. L. (2011). Successful implementation of new technologies in nursing care: A questionnaire survey of nurse-users. BMC Medical Informatics and Decision Making, 11(67), 1–12.

Joffe, S. W., Webster, K., McManus, D. D., Kiernan, M. S., Lessard, D., Yarzebski, J., … Goldberg, R. J. (2013). Improved survival after heart failure: A community-based perspective. Journal of the American Heart Association, 2(3), 1–9. doi: 10.1161/JAHA.113.000053

Jones, C. L., Jensen, J. D., Scherr, C. L., Brown, N. R., Christy, K., & Weaver, J. (2015). The Health Belief Model as an explanatory framework in communication research: Exploring parallel, serial, and moderated mediation. Health Communication, 30(6), 566–576.

James, J. (2013). Patient engagement. Health Affairs Health Policy Brief. Retrieved from https://www.healthaffairs.org/do/10.1377/hpb20130214.898775/full/. doi: 10.1377/hpb20130214.898775

Kennard, D. K. (2016). Health literacy concepts in nursing education. Nursing Education Perspectives, 37(2), 118–119.

Knapp, H. (2017). Practical statistics for nursing using SPSS. Thousand Oaks, CA: Sage. Knapp, T. R. (2016). Why is the one-group pretest-posttest design still used? Clinical Nursing Research, 25(5), 467–472. doi:10.1177/1054773816666280

Koh, H. K., Brach, C., Harris, L. M., & Parchman, M. L. (2013). A proposed health literate care model would constitute a systems approach to improving patient engagement in care. Health Affairs, 32(2), 357–367.

Kollia, Z. A., Giakoumidakis, K., & Brokalaki, H. (2016). The effectiveness of nursing education on clinical outcomes of patients with heart failure: A systematic review. Chronic Disease Care, 5(2), 1–11.

Kutner, M., Greenberg, E., Jin, Y., & Paulsen, C. (2006). The health literacy of America's adults: Results from the 2003 national assessment of adult literacy. US Department of Education. Washington, DC: National Center for Educational Statistics.

Lambert, V., & Keogh, D. (2014). Health literacy and its importance for effective communication. Part 1. Nursing Children and Young People, 26(3), 31–37. doi:10.7748/ncyp2014.04.26.3.31e387

Latimer, N. (2018). How technology is shaping patient education. Retrieved from https://www.cerner.com/blog/how-technology-is-shaping-patient-education

LaVela, S. L., & Gallan, A. S. (2014). Evaluation and measurement of patient experience. Patient Experiences Journal, 1(1), 27–36.

Lessa, Q. C. S. S., Frossard, J. D. M., Santos, F. A. S., Queluci, G. C., Correia, D. M. S., & Cavalcanti, A. C. D. (2016). Nursing actions for patients with heart failure: an integrative review. Journal of Respiratory Care Online, 8(2), 4587–4600.

Levy, H., Janke, A. T., & Langa, K.M. (2015). Health literacy and the digital divide among older Americans. Journal of Geriatric Internal Medicine, 30(3), 284–289. doi: 10.1007/s11606-014-3069-5

Liu, Y., Avant, K. C., Aungsuroch, Y., Zhang, X., & Jiang, P. (2014). Patient outcomes in the field of nursing: A concept analysis. International Journal of Nursing Science, 1(1), 69–74.

Logan, R. A., Wong, W. F., Villaire, M., Daus, G., Parnell, T. A., Willis, E., … Paasche-Orlow, M. K. (2015). Health literacy: A necessary element for achieving health equity. Washington, DC: Institute of Medicine. Discussion Paper. Retrieved from https://nam.edu/wp-content/uploads/2015/07/NecessaryElement.pdf

Mackert, M., Mabry-Flynn, A., Champlin, S., Donovan, E. E., & Pounders, K. (2016). Health literacy and health information technology adoption: The potential for a new digital divide. Journal of Medical Internet Research, 18(10), 1–19. doi: 10.2196/jmir.6349

MacLeod, S., Musich, S., Gulyas, S., Cheng, Y., Tkatch, R., Cempellin, D., … Yeh, C. S. (2017). The impact of inadequate health literacy on patient satisfaction, healthcare utilization, and expenditures among older adults. Geriatric Nursing, 38, 334–341.

Matsuoka, S., Tsuchihashi-Makaya, M., Kayane, T., Yamada, M., Wakabayashi, R., Kato, N. P., & Yazawa, M. (2016). Health literacy is independently associated with self-care behavior in patients with heart failure. Patient Education and Counseling, 99(6), 1026–1032. doi: 10.1016/j.pec.2016.01.003

McCormack, L., Thomas, V., Lewis, M. A., & Rudd, R. (2016). Improving low health literacy and patient engagement: A social ecological approach. Patient Education and Counseling, 100, 8–13.

McCrum-Gardner, E. (2010). Sample size and power calculations made simple. International Journal of Therapy and Rehabilitation, 17(1), 10–14.

McLeod, S. A. (2013). What is validity? Retrieved from https://www.simplypsychology.org/validity.html

McLeod, S. A. (2017). What's the difference between qualitative and quantitative research? Retrieved from https://www.simplypsychology.org/qualitative-quantitative.html

Meade, S., & Pierce, B. (2016). Using new technology to improve patient experiences. ASQ's Healthcare Update, 1–3.

Melnyk, B. M. (2012). The role of technology in enhancing evidence-based practice, education, healthcare quality, and patient outcomes: A call for randomized controlled trials and comparative effectiveness research. Worldviews on Evidence-Based Nursing, 63–65.

Meng, K., Seekatz, B., Haug, G., Mosler, G., Schwaab, B., Worringen, U., & Faller, H. (2014). Evaluation of a standardized patient education program for inpatient cardiac rehabilitation: Impact on illness knowledge and self-management behaviors up to 1 year. Health Education Research, 29(2), 235–246.

Mocean, F., Lotrean, L., Lorena, F., & Baritz, M. (2009). Using modern information technology in health promotion through various forms of health education at community. Mathematical Methods and Applied Computing, 458–462.

Mosen, D. M., Schmittdiel, J., Hibbard, J., Sobel, D., Remmers, C., & Bellows, J. (2007). Is patient activation associated with outcomes of care for adults with chronic conditions? Journal of Ambulatory Care Management, 30(1), 21–29.

Nieswiadomy, R. M. (2012). Foundations of Nursing Research (6th ed.). Upper Saddle River, NJ: Pearson Education.

Nijhawan, L., Janodia, M., Muddukrishna, B., Bhat, K., Bairy, K., N. Udupa, N., & Musmade, P. (2013). Informed consent: Issues and challenges. Journal of Advanced Pharmaceutical Technology & Research, 4(3), 134–140. doi: 10.4103/2231-4040.116779

Nunlist, M. M., Blumberg, J., Uiterwyk, S., Apgar, T. (2016). Using health confidence to improve patient outcomes. Family Practice Management, 23(6), 21–24.

Nuzzo, R. (2018). Tips for communicating statistical significance. Retrieved from https://www.nih.gov/about-nih/what-we-do/science-health-public-trust/perspectives/science-health-public-trust/tips-communicating-statistical-significance

Office of Disease Prevention and Health Promotion (2010). National action plan to improve health literacy. Retrieved from https://health.gov/communication/HLActionPlan/pdf/Health_Literacy_Action_Plan.pdf

Office of Disease Prevention & Health Promotion. (2017a). Health communication and health information technology. Retrieved from https://www.healthypeople.gov/2020/topics-objectives/topic/health-communication-and-health-information-technology

Office of Disease Prevention & Health Promotion. (2017b). Disparities. Retrieved from https://www.healthypeople.gov/2020/about/foundation-health-measures/Disparities

Office of Disease Prevention & Health Promotion. (2017c). National action plan to improve health literacy. Retrieved from https://health.gov/communication/initiatives/health-literacy-action-plan.asp

Office of Disease Prevention and Health Promotion. (2018). National action plan to improve health literacy. Retrieved from https://health.gov/communication/initiatives/health-literacy-action-plan.asp

Office of Disease Prevention and Health Promotion. (2019a). Social determinants of health. Retrieved from https://www.healthypeople.gov/2020/topics-objectives/topic/social-determinants-of-health/objectives

Office of Disease Prevention and Health Promotion. (2019b). Health communication and health information technology. Retrieved from https://www.healthypeople.gov/node/3508/objectives#4513

Office of the National Coordinator for Health Information Technology. (2018). Patient education and engagement. Retrieved from https://www.healthit.gov/topic/patient-education-and-engagement

Orem, D. E. (1995). Nursing Concepts of practice (5th ed.). Philadelphia: Mosby.

Orem, D. (2001). Nursing Concepts of practice (6th ed.). Philadelphia: Mosby.

Orem, D. E., & Taylor, S. G. (2011). Reflections on nursing practice science: The nature, the structure, and the foundation of nursing sciences. Nursing Science Quarterly, 24(1), 35–41. doi: 10.1177/0894318410389061

Pannucci, C. J. & Wilkins, E. G. (2010). Identifying and avoiding bias in research. Plastic and Reconstructive Surgery, 126(2), 619–625.

Paterick, T. E., Patel, N., Tajik, A. J., Chandrasekaran, K. (2017). Improving health outcomes through patient education and partnerships with patients. Baylor University Medical Center Proceedings, 30(1), 112–113.

Patmon, F. L., Gee, P. M., Rylee, T. L., & Readdy, N. L. (2016). Using interactive patient engagement technology in clinical practice: A Qualitative assessment of nurses' perceptions. Journal of Medical Internet Research, 18(11), 1–10.

Peterson, P. N., Shetterly, S. M., Clarke, C. L., Bekelman, D. B., Chan, P. S., Allen, L. A., … Masoudi, F. A. (2011). Health literacy and outcomes among patients with heart failure. JAMA: The Journal of the American Medical Association, 305(16), 1695–1701. doi: 10.1001/jama.2011.512

Pourhoseingholi, M. A., Baghestani, A. R., & Vahedi, M. (2012). How to control confounding effects by statistical analysis. Gastroenterology and Hepatology from Bed to Bench, 5(2), 79–83.

Prey, J. E., Qian, M., Restaino, S., Hibbard, J., Bakken, S., Schnall, R., … Creber, R. M. (2016). Reliability and validity of the patient activation measure in hospitalized patients. Patient Education and Counseling, 99(12), 2026–2033.

Prey, J. E., Woollen, J., Wilcox, L., Sackeim, A., Hripcsak, G., Bakken, S., Restaino, S., … Vawdrey, D. K. (2014). Patient engagement in the inpatient setting: a systematic review. Journal of American Medical Informatics Association, 21(4), 742–750.

Price, P. C., Jhangiani, R. S., & Chiang, C. A. (2015). Research Methods in Psychology. Retrieved from https://opentextbc.ca/researchmethods/

Rebar, C. R., Gersch, C. J., Macnee, C. L., and McCabe, S. (2010). Understanding nursing research: Reading and using research in evidence-based practice (3rd ed.). Philadelphia, PA: Lippincott, Williams, and Wilkins.

Riley, J. (2015). Key roles for the nurse in acute heart failure management. Cardiac Failure Review, 1(2), 123–127. doi: 10.15420/cfr.2015.1.2.123

Romain, P. L. (2015). Conflicts of interest in research: Looking out for number one means keeping the primary interest front and center. Current Reviews in Musculoskeletal Medicine, 8(2), 122–127. doi: 10.1007/s12178-015-9270-2

Rowe, J. (2013). Ethics or innovation: Which comes first? Retrieved from http://www.healthcareitnews.com/blog/ethics-or-innovation-which-comes-first

Rouleau, G., Gagnon, M. P., & Cote, J. (2015). Impacts of information and communication technologies on nursing care: An overview of systematic reviews (protocols). Systematic Reviews, 4. doi: 10.1186/s13643-015-0062y

Rumsey, D. (2016). How to interpret a correlation coefficient R. Retrieved from https://www.dummies.com/education/math/statistics/how-to-interpret-a-correlation-coefficient-r/

Ryan, P. (2009). Integrated theory of health behavior change. Clinical Nurse Specialist, 23(3), 161–172.

Rymer, J. A., Kaltenbach, L. A., Anstrom, K. J., Fonarow, G. C., Erskine, N., Peterson, E. D., … Wang, T. Y. (2018). Hospital evaluation of health literacy and associated outcomes in patients after acute myocardial infarction. American Heart Journal, 198, 97–107. doi: 10.1016/j.ahj.2017.08.024

Sacristán, J. A., Aguarón, A., Avendaño-Solá, C., Garrido, P., Carrión, J., Guiérrez, A., … Flores, A. (2016). Patient involvement in clinical research: why, when, and how. Patient Preference and Adherence, 10, 631–640. doi: 10.2147/PPA.S104259

Sahlsten, M. J. M., Larsson, I. E., Sjöström, B., & Plos, K. A. E. (2008). An analysis of the concept of patient participation. Nursing Forum, 43(1), 2–11. Retrieved from https://doi.org/10.1111/j.1744-6198.2008.00090.x

Schillinger, D., Grumbach, K., & Piette, J. (2002). Association of health literacy with diabetes outcomes. JAMA: The Journal of American Medicine, 288(4), 475–482. doi:10.1001/jama.288.4.475

Shigaki, C. L., Kruse, R. L., Mehr, D. R., & Ge, B. (2012). The REALM vs. NVS: A comparison of health literacy measures in patients with diabetes. Annals of Behavioral Science and Medical Education, 18(1), 9–13.

Skelly, A. C., Dettori, J. R., & Brodt, E. D. (2012). Assessing bias: The importance of considering confounding. Evidence-Based Spine-Care Journal, 3(1), 9–12.

Skolasky, R. L., Green, A. F., Scharfstein, D., Boult, C., Reider, L., & Wegener, S. T. (2011). Psychometric properties of the patient activation measure among multimorbid older adults. Health Research and Educational Trust, 46(2), 457–478.

Smith, S. G., Curtis, L. M., Wardle, J., von Wagner, C., & Wolf, M. S. (2013). Skill set or mind set? Associations between health literacy, patient activation and health. PLOS ONE, 8(9), 1–7.

Smith, S. G., Jackson, S. E., Kobayashi, L. C., & Steptoe, A. (2018). Social isolation, health literacy, and mortality risk: Findings from the English longitudinal study of ageing. Health Psychology, 37(2), 160–169. doi: 10.1037/hea0000541

Solomon, M. R. (2014). Is information technology making a difference in engaging patients? Journal of Healthcare Information Management, 28(1), Retrieved from www.himss.org/jhim/archive/volume-28-2014

Sorensen, K., Van den Broucke, S., Fullam, J., Doyle, G., Pelikan, J., Slonska, Z., Brand, H., & HLS-EU Consortium Health Literacy Project European. (2012). Health literacy and public health: A systematic review and integration of definitions and models. BMC Public Health, 12, 80. doi: 10.1186/1471-2458-12-80

Stagliano, V., & Wallace, L. S. (2013). Brief health literacy screening items predict newest vital sign scores. Journal of the American Board of Family Medicine, 26(5), 558–565. doi: 10.3122/jabfm.2013.05.130096

Sudore, R. L., Yaffe, S., Satterfield, S., Harris, T. B., Mehta, K. M., Simonsick, A. B., … Schilinger, D. (2006). Limited literacy and mortality in the elderly: The heat, aging, and body composition study. Journal of General Internal Medicine, 21(8), 806–812.

Sullivan, G. M. (2011). A primer on the validity of assessment instruments. Journal of Graduate Medical Education 3(2), 119–120. doi: 10.4300/JGME-D-11-00075.1

The Health Information Management Systems Society. (2019). What is patient engagement? Retrieved from https://www.himss.org/library/patient-engagement-toolkit

The National Commission for the Protection of Human Subjects of Biomedical and Behavioral Research. (1979). The Belmont Report. Obtained from https://www.hhs.gov/ohrp/sites/default/files/the-belmont-report-508c_FINAL.pdf

Thompson, C. J. (2017). What's the difference between statistical significance and clinical significance? Retrieved from https://nursingeducationexpert.com/difference-statistical-significance-clinical-significance/

Thornton, I., & Hipskind, J. E. (2019). Informed consent. Retrieved from https://www.ncbi.nlm.nih.gov/books/NBK430827/#_NBK430827_pubdet_

Toscos, T., Daley, C., Heral, L., Doshi, R., Chen, Y. C., Eckert, G. J., … Mirro, M. J. (2016). Impacts of electronic personal health record use on engagement and intermediate health outcomes among cardiac patients: a quasi-experimental study. Journal of American Medical Informatics Association, 23(1), 119–128. doi: 10.1093/jamia/ocv164

Tsai, A. C., Morton, S. C., Mangione, C. M., & Keeler, E. B. (2005). A meta-analysis of interventions to improve care for chronic illnesses. The American Journal of Managed Care, 11(8), 478–488.

U.S. Department of Health & Human Services. (2017). Health information technology. Retrieved from https://www.hhs.gov/hipaa/for-professionals/special-topics/health-information-technology/index.html

U.S. Office of Disease Prevention and Health Promotion. (2010). National Action Plan to Improve Health Literacy. Washington, DC: Author.

U.S. Department of Health & Human Services. (2016). Health Literacy Measurement Tools (Revised). Retrieved from https://www.ahrq.gov/professionals/quality-patient-safety/quality-resources/tools/literacy/index.html

U. S. Department of Education. (2019). National Assessment of Adult Literacy (NAAL): Health literacy. Retrieved from https://nces.ed.gov/naal/health.asp

U.S. Department of Health & Human Services. (2008). America's health literacy: Why we need accessible health information. An issue brief from the U. S. Department of Health and Human Services. Retrieved from https://health.gov/communication/literacy/issuebrief/

U.S. Office of Disease Prevention and Health Promotion. (2010). National Action Plan to Improve Health Literacy. Washington, DC: Author. Retrieved from https://health.gov/communication/initiatives/health-literacy-action-plan.asp

Vadillo, M. A., Konstantinidis, E., & Shanks, D. R. (2016). Underpowered samples, false negatives, and unconscious learning. Psychonomic Bulletin & Review, 23, 87–102. doi: 10.3758/s13423-015-0892-6

Vahey, D., Aiken, L., Sloane, D., Clarke, S., & Vargas, D. (2004). Nurse burnout and patient satisfaction. Medical Care, 42(2) supplement, 57–66.

Vernon, J. A., Trujillo, A., Rosenbaum, S., & DeBuono, B. (2007). Low health literacy: Implications for national health policy. Retrieved from https://publichealth.gwu.edu/departments/healthpolicy/CHPR/downloads/LowHealthLiteracyReport10_4_07.pdf

Villarruel, A. M., Bishop, T. L., Simpson, E. M., Jemmott, L. S., & Fawcett, J. (2001). Borrowed theories, shared theories, and the advancement of nursing knowledge. Nursing Science Quarterly, 14(2), 158–163.

Wasson, J., & Coleman, E. A. (2014). Health confidence: A simple, essential measure for patient engagement and better practice. Family Practice Management, 21(5), 8–12.

Waters, J. (2017). Correlational research guidelines: Conducting correlational research. Retrieved from https://www.capilanou.ca/programs-courses/psychology/student

Weiss, B. D., Mays, M. Z., Martz, W., Castro, K. M., DeWalt, D., Pignone, M. P., … Hale, F. A. (2005). Quick assessment of literacy in primary care: The newest vital sign. Annals of Family Medicine, 3(6), 514–522. doi: 10.1370/afam.405

Werder, M. (2015). Health information technology: A key ingredient of the patient experience. Patient Experience Journal, 2(1), 143–147.

White, M., Garbez, R., Carroll, M., Brinker, E., & Howie-Esquivel, J. (2013). Is teach-back associated with knowledge retention and hospital readmission in hospitalized heart failure patients? Journal of Cardiovascular Nursing, 28(2), 137–146. doi: 10.1097/JCN. 0b013e31824987bd

White, M. F., Kirschner, J., & Hamilton, M. A. (2014). Self-care guide for the heart failure patient. American Heart Association Journals, 129, e293-e294.

White, S. (2008). Assessing the nation's health literacy: Key concepts and findings of the National Assessment of Adult Literacy (NAAL). Chicago, IL: American Medical Association. Retrieved from http://s3.amazonaws.com/zanran_storage/www.ama-assn.org/ContentPages/11339828.pdf

Whittaker, G. S. (2015). An educational approach for "non-compliant" patients. The Canadian Journal of Critical Care Nursing, 26(3), 11–15.

Wickham, C. A., & Carbone, E. T. (2013). Can technology improve health literacy? Journal of Nutritional Disorders and Therapy, 3(3), 1–2. doi:10.4172/2161-0509.1000e114

Wilson, F. L., Baker, L. M., Nordstrom, C. K., & Legwand, C. (2008). Using the teach-back and Orem's self-care deficit nursing theory to increase childhood immunization communication among low-income mothers. Issues in Comprehensive Pediatric Nursing, 31(7), 7–22.

Wilson, F. L., Mayeta-Peart, A., Parada-Webster, L., & Nordstrom, C. (2012). Using the teach-back method to increase maternal immunization literacy among low-income pregnant women in Jamaica: A pilot study. Journal of Pediatric Nursing, 27, 451–459.

Wilson, F. L., Mood, D. W., Risk, J., & Kershaw, T. (2003). Evaluation of education materials using Orem's self-care deficit theory. Nursing Science Quarterly, 16(1), 68–76. doi: 10.1177/0894318402239069

Wittenberg, E., Ferrell, B., Kanter, E., & Buller, H. (2018). Health literacy: Exploring nursing challenges to providing support and understanding. Clinical Journal of Oncology Nursing, 22(1), 53–61.

Wittink, H., & Oosterhaven, J. (2018). Patient education and health literacy. Musculoskeletal Science and Practice, 38, 120–127. doi: 10.1016/j.msksp.2018.06.004

Wolf, M. S., & Bailey, S. C. (2009). The role of health literacy in patient safety. Retrieved from https://psnet.ahrq.gov/perspectives/perspective/72/the-role-of-health-literacy-in-patient-safety

World Health Organization. (2016). Patient engagement: Technical series on safer primary care. Retrieved from https://apps.who.int/iris/bitstream/handle/10665/252269/9789241511629-eng.pdf;jsessionid=BC09F42820712BD46C5765686181A570?sequence=1

Yin, S. H., Johnson, M., Mendelsohn, A. L., Abrams, M. A., Sanders, L. M., & Dreyer, B. P. (2009). The health literacy of parents in the United States: A nationally representative study. Pediatrics, 124(3), 289–298.

Zan, S., Agboola, S., Moore, S. A., Parks, K. A., Kvedar, J. C., Jethwani, K. (2015). Patient engagement with a mobile web-based telemonitoring system for heart failure self-management: A pilot study. JMIR Mhealth Uhealth, 3(2), 1–14. doi: 10.2196/mhealth.3789

Zare, M., Ghodsbin, F., Jahanbin, I., Ariafar, A., Keshavarzi, S., & Izadi, T. (2016). The effect of health belief model-based education on knowledge and prostate cancer screening behaviors: A randomized controlled trial. International Journal of Community Based Nursing and Midwifery, 4(1), 57–68.

APPENDIX A

IRB Approval Letter

GRAND CANYON UNIVERSITY

3300 West Camelback Road, Phoenix Arizona 85017 602.639.7500 Toll Free 800.800.9776 www.gcu.edu

DATE:	November 27, 2018
TO:	Melissa Sorgeloos
FROM:	Grand Canyon University Institutional Review Board
STUDY TITLE:	Does Health Literacy Influence Patient Use of Interactive Patient Engagement Technology (iPET) Within the Acute Care Setting?
IRB REFERENCE #:	IRB-2018-616
SUBMISSION TYPE:	Initial Review Submission Packet
ACTION:	Determination of Exempt Status
DECISION DATE:	November 27, 2018
REVIEW CATEGORY:	N/A

Thank you for your submission of New Project materials for this research study.

GCU is not the IRB of record since prior IRB approval was obtained from IRB. IRB: Expedited Review status obtained on October 31, 2018.

Grand Canyon University Institutional Review Board has determined this project is EXEMPT FROM IRB REVIEW according to federal regulations. You now have GCU IRB approval to collect data.

If applicable, please use the approved informed consent that is included in your published documents.

We will put a copy of this correspondence on file in our office.

If you have any questions, please contact the IRB office at irb@gcu.edu or 602-639-7804. Please include your study title and reference number in all correspondence with this office.

Cynthia Bainbridge

Dr. Cynthia Bainbridge
Assistant Dean, Research and Dissertations Director, Institutional Review Board College of Doctoral Studies

APPENDIX B

REALM-SF Scoresheet – Assessor Version

REALM-SF Score Sheet

ID:________ Date:________ Birth year:____________ Gender:_______

- ❑ **Behavior**
- ❑ **Exercise**
- ❑ **Menopause**
- ❑ **Rectal**
- ❑ **Antibiotics**
- ❑ **Anemia**
- ❑ **Jaundice**

TOTAL SCORE = ______ (❑= 1)

iPET used: Education

❑ YES

❑ NO

Scores and Grade Equivalents for the REALM-SF

Score	Grade range/Educational Considerations
0	Third grade and below; will not be able to read most low-literacy materials; will need repeated oral instructions, materials composed primarily of illustrations, or audio or video tapes.
1-3	Fourth to sixth grade; will need low-literacy materials, may not be able to read prescription labels.
4-6	Seventh to eighth grade; will struggle with most patient education materials; will not be offended by low-literacy materials.
7	High school; will be able to read most patient education materials.

APPENDIX C

REALM-SF Tool – Patient Version

REALM-SF

In health care, doctors and nurses often use words that patients do not understand. I am looking at words that doctors and nurses often use with their patients in order to improve communication between health care providers and patients.

Here is a list of medical words.

Starting at the top of the list, please read each word aloud to me. If you do not recognize a word, you can say 'pass' and move on to the next word.

- ☐ Behavior
- ☐ Exercise
- ☐ Menopause
- ☐ Rectal
- ☐ Antibiotics
- ☐ Anemia
- ☐ Jaundice

APPENDIX D

REALM-SF Use Approval

From: Davis, Terry
To: Sorgeloos, Melissa - PHX
Subject: Re: Permission for use of REALM-SF tool
Date: Wednesday, June 20, 2018 11:50:16 AM
Attachments: mo info.txt

Melissa
You have my permission to use REALM sf.

Good luck w your cool project
Terry

Sent from my iPhone

On Jun 20, 2018, at 1:30 PM, Sorgeloos, Melissa - PHX
<Melissa.Sorgeloos@> wrote:

EXTERNAL EMAIL: EVALUATE

Hello Dr. Davis,

Greetings.

I am a doctoral student in the Doctor of Nursing practice program at Grand Canyon University. I am conducting my direct practice improvement project on health literacy and the correlation between patient use of technology, in particular the interactive patient engagement technology (iPET) at the

I seek to discover if patients with higher health literacy scores tend to be more apt to partake in the use of healthcare related technology for educational purposes while hospitalized in an acute care hospital setting.

I am writing to you to obtain permission to use the Rapid Estimate of Adult Literacy in Medicine – Short Form (REALM-SF). I would be happy to answer any questions you have about my project.

Thank you for your time and consideration.

Have a great day!

Melissa Sorgeloos, MSN, RN, MBA

APPENDIX E

iPET Guide for Patients

Instructions for Using Your Remote

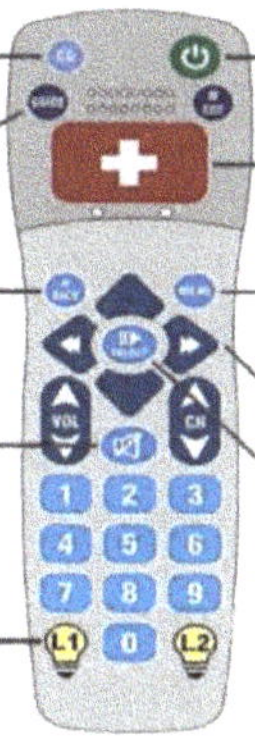

CLOSED CAPTIONING Display text

TV GUIDE See what's on TV

BACK Return to previous menu

MUTE Turn sound ON and OFF

LIGHTS Turn lights ON and OFF

POWER Turn TV ON and OFF

NURSE CALL Call for a Nurse

MENU Interactive Health Care Programming Main Menu

ARROWS Use to move through menu

SELECT Use to select a menu choice

PAUSING, SKIPPING, AND REPLAYING VIDEOS

While a video is playing, use the SELECT button to pause, then use the right and left directional buttons to skip forward or backward and to replay.

PLEASE NOTE: Skip forward is not available on educational videos.

iPET System

From the MAIN MENU, here are the system options:

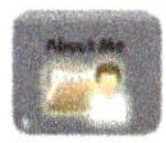

Review the details of your care

My Education Learn more about your condition

My Allergies Confirm your allergy list

My Medication Review your list of home medications

Discharge Planning Things to do before you leave

Today's Menu See what we're preparing for you

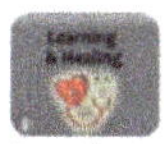

Discover the ways we support your mind, body and spirit

Video Library Learn about a variety of medical conditions

Medication Library Read up on common medications

Spiritual Services Request support from spiritual services

My Health Online Receive helpful health management tips after you leave

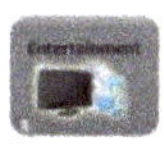

Enjoy programming from movies to gentle relaxation

Watch TV Don't miss your favorite programs

Movies Hits and family-friendly films

Relaxation Restful sounds and images

Spiritual Programming to soothe the soul

Noise Suppression Ambient sound reduces distractions

Music Tunes Offering a variety of eras and genres

Sleep Timer Timer automatically turns off TV

Parental Control PIN code restricts movie categories

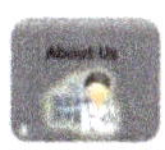

Learn more about our hospital and services

Patient Guide Everything you need to know from admission to discharge

Hospital Information Our programs, services, and hours

APPENDIX F

Health Literacy and Patient use of iPET

SCRIPT FOR PATIENT PARTICIPATION

You are eligible to participate in this project study if you are age 18 years or older and are able to speak and read English.

You are not eligible to participate in this project if you are under the age of 18 years or are over the age of 89 years. You are also not eligible if you are unable to speak and read English, as the study tool is only available in English.

About 50 people will be asked to take part in this project and if you choose to take part in this study, I will:

1. Ask you the year you were born.
2. Ask you your identifiable gender.
3. Ask you to read seven one-word medical terms aloud to me.

If you decide to participate in this voluntary project study, you may face some minimal risks. Risks related to participation may include the potential to experience minor anxiety, as many patients may not be comfortable reading medical terms aloud.

To decrease the impact of these risks, you can choose not to participate. You can decide to stop participation at any time during my time with you today. If you decide to opt out or not participate today, there will not be any consequences for withdrawal from this study.

In addition to the risks described above, there may be unknown risks, or risks that we did not anticipate, associated with being in this voluntary project study.

If you decide to participate today, there will be no direct benefit to you from taking part in this study. However, it is hoped that the information gained from the study will help in the treatment of future patients with conditions like yours. Participation in this study will not cause you to give you up your legal rights. Your treatment and care will not be affected by your decision to or to not participate. It is not anticipated, but under some circumstances, an unanticipated circumstance may cause me to end your participation in this voluntary project study.

Your records will remain confidential. I will not be collecting any confidential information from you. I will not have access to your chart or medical record. Your name will not be collected. I will assign you an anonymous study number, which cannot be traced back to you.

There are no conflicts of interest with your participation today and there is no funding for this project study. [illegible], Grand Canyon University and the team are receiving no payments from other agencies, organizations, or companies to conduct this research study. You will not be paid for taking part in this voluntary project study.

You will not incur any costs for participating in this project study. You or your medical/hospital insurance carrier will remain responsible for your regular medical care expenses. This study will not provide any payments or compensation for any expenses incurred during your hospitalization.

I encourage you to ask questions. If you have any questions about the research study itself, please free to ask me at this time. I would be happy to answer any questions that you may have.

Should you have any questions about your rights as a voluntary project study participant, you may call the Institutional Review Board, which is concerned with protection of volunteers in research projects. I have printed their information for you.

**(Will provide the patient with IRB information in written format)

www.ingramcontent.com/pod-product-compliance
Lightning Source LLC
LaVergne TN
LVHW050914210926
848482LV00012B/435